Biotechne: Interthinking Art, Science And Design

Biotechne: Interthinking Art, Science and Design publishes books about the history, theory, and practice of art and design as they comingle with the natural sciences. The series title reclaims the Greek meanings of the roots bios, conveying life, the living, or citizen-life, and techne, conveying art, skill, or craft. Biotechne thus names the folding of "art" and "science" into complex and hybrid practices that transcend a human-centered "engineering" worldview. "Interthinking," a neologism invented by art and science visionary György Kepes, describes knowledge informed by ecological, systemic, and cybernetic connections, defining the active engagement among fields central to the Biotechne series. This engagement is the source of the cultural creativity and resourcefulness necessary to thrive in the rapidly changing world conditions of the Anthropocene. Biotechne welcomes proposals treating art and design subjects from any time period, antiquity to the present, which speak directly to these contemporary concerns. We seek inventive, cross-pollinating works about the arts and their engagement with sciences from astrobiology to zoology, wherever that engagement occurs, in art or design studios, scientific laboratories, natural habitats, the museum and gallery worlds, performance spaces, medical practices, and the political realm. By identifying significant intersections of art, humanities, and science, and tracking rigorous paths through the cross-disciplinary information jungle, Biotechne serves audiences of both experts and lay readers while substantiating the role of aesthetic insight within the natural sciences.

Titles in the Series

D'Arcy Wentworth Thompson's Generative Influences in Art, Design, and Architecture: From Forces to Forms, edited by Ellen K. Levy and Charissa N. Terranova (2021)

Sea Currents in Nineteenth-Century Art, Science and Culture: Commodifying the Ocean World, edited by Molly Duggins and Kathleen Davidson (2023)

Plants by Numbers: Art, Computation and Queer Feminist Technoscience, edited by Helen V. Pritchard and Jane Prophet (2023)

Space Feminisms: People, Planets, Power, edited by Marie-Pier Boucher, Claire Webb, Annick Bureaud, and Nahum (2024)

Art and Biotechnology: Viral Culture from CRISPR to COVID, edited by Claire Nettleton and Louise Mackenzie (2024)

Viral Behaviors

Viruses and Viral Phenomena across Science, Technology, and the Arts

Roberta Buiani

BLOOMSBURY VISUAL ARTS
LONDON • NEW YORK • OXFORD • NEW DELHI • SYDNEY

BLOOMSBURY VISUAL ARTS
Bloomsbury Publishing Plc
50 Bedford Square, London, WC1B 3DP, UK
1385 Broadway, New York, NY 10018, USA
29 Earlsfort Terrace, Dublin 2, Ireland

BLOOMSBURY, BLOOMSBURY VISUAL ARTS and the Diana logo are
trademarks of Bloomsbury Publishing Plc

First published in Great Britain 2024

Cover design: Elena Durey
Cover image: Elaine Whittaker, *Pandemic Convergence* 1/2, 2020.
Acrylic on Paper © Elaine Whittaker

A catalogue record for this book is available from the British Library.

Library of Congress Cataloging-in-Publication Data
Names: Buiani, Roberta, author.
Title: Viral behaviors : viruses and viral phenomena across science,
technology, and the arts / Roberta Buiani.
Description: London : Bloomsbury Visual Arts, 2024. |
Series: Biotechne: interthinking art, science and design ; [vol 6] |
Includes bibliographical references and index.
Identifiers: LCCN 2023058309 (print) | LCCN 2023058310 (ebook) |
ISBN 9781350419421 (hardback) | ISBN 9781350419469 (paperback) |
ISBN 9781350419438 (pdf) | ISBN 9781350419445 (ebook)
Subjects: LCSH: Science and the arts. | Arts and society. | Viruses.
Classification: LCC NX180.S3 B85 2024 (print) | LCC NX180.S3 (ebook) |
DDC 700/.4561–dc23/eng/20240403
LC record available at https://lccn.loc.gov/2023058309
LC ebook record available at https://lccn.loc.gov/2023058310

ISBN: HB: 978-1-3504-1942-1
ePDF: 978-1-3504-1943-8
eBook: 978-1-3504-1944-5

Series: Biotechne: Interthinking Art, Science and Design

Typeset by Integra Software Services Pvt. Ltd.
Printed and bound in Great Britain

To find out more about our authors and books visit www.bloomsbury.com
and sign up for our newsletters.

To those who have dared to embrace the viral

CONTENTS

ILLUSTRATIONS

Introduction

It was June 2017. While I was visiting the fifty-seventh Biennale di Venezia, an installation at the Danish Pavilion drew my attention. The installation was titled *Influenza, Theatre of Glowing Darkness*, by artist Kirstine Roepstorff (Roepstorff 2017; "Venice Biennale 2017 Archive" 2017). The term influenza stands for the verb "to influence" and for the viral infection that visits us every year. The interdisciplinary installation extended beyond the space of the pavilion and merged with the surrounding Giardini. Visitors were then directed into a pitch-dark room and guided to sit on stools located around a rectangular perimeter. Then the show started. The room was softly lit by a scheme of lights that reflected and bounced around through what seemed like a maze of glasses. The light was subtle, purposely faint, and hardly visible, as participants struggled to grasp the scene from their seats. Roepstorff clearly wanted participants to experience darkness, not as a fearful, indeterminate space, but as a strange place, where initial disorientation makes room for a marvelous, if uncomfortable, curiosity. Here are the first words introducing the show:

> Darkness.
> When everything was just floating energy in complete darkness …
> Maybe you remember which choices you made here?
> How much did you dare to risk in order to grow?
> How much darkness did you absorb?
> Do you remember?

Built as a dialogue between a seed impatient to grow and to burst out of its protective membrane, a dark river, and a midwife recounting a painful experience of loss and recovery, the short play that followed asked the participants to reflect on aspects that seem in opposition but are clearly two sides of the same coin. Traditionally, darkness is perceived as the opposite of light; light metaphorically stands for vision and knowledge. Fear of darkness is associated with fear of the unknown: in the past, when roads were unlit, and mysterious miasma was believed to take human beings without apparent reasons, darkness was certainly an unwelcome presence (Bauman 2006). Roepstorff asks us to question these commonplaces. When the world goes dark, how do we react? By associating influenza with the fear of the unknown, and by proposing that instead of becoming overwhelmed by fear we start looking inside darkness for elements that can produce growth and renewal, Roepstorff made me reflect. Was she inviting me to embrace the unknown?

We are all familiar with viruses and their reputation. As the most abundant biological agents on earth, viruses are "small obligate intracellular parasites, which by definition contain either a RNA or DNA genome surrounded by a protective, virus-coded protein coat" (Gelderblom 1996). Viruses can be found attached to cells, to bacteria (bacteriophages), and even to other viruses (virophages). Viruses are often innocuous to humans and animals, but a few of them are known to cause harm. This is sufficient to fear and antagonize them. During the 1970s, the realm of computing defined another category of viruses: computer viruses. These digital self-replicating strings of code enter and modify a host operating system, causing a chain reaction, and potentially disrupting entire networks and the liveliness of those who depend on their smooth functioning.

Whether informational or biological, viruses appear to possess shared qualities. In fact, the immateriality of viruses and their non-linear and relational behavior have puzzled scientists and digital information experts: as biological viruses are submicroscopic, computer viruses are constituted by code. In both cases, they do not exist as self-contained entities, but entangled with their hosts and their surrounding environment. Interestingly, these qualities extend across realms, disciplines, and contexts. They are not limited to the specificity of one biological entity or one self-replicating agent but belong to the collective assemblage of all contagious phenomena. The same qualities are attributed to a set of trends and practices. Viruses produce a great deal of emotional responses; they are defined by a variety of stereotypical connotations. These attributes, too, cross disciplinary boundaries. All these qualities, material and metaphorical, emotional and stereotypical, converge into the *viral*.

I use the term viral as an overarching category emphasizing a series of features carried by viruses (e.g., their seemingly unpredictable behavior, their complicated intersection with the surrounding environment and their host, their status as partially alive, etc.). Thanks to a variety of processes of simplification (e.g., the idea that viral videos spread like ... viruses), these features have become the subjects of appropriations and imitations. As a result, viruses have proliferated beyond delimited scientific and technological areas of competence, to easily circulate across and to be absorbed by digital media, popular culture, and the arts. These processes effectively demonstrate the propensity of viruses to spread in a transdisciplinary fashion and reveal the complicated connections that shape them and that they generate.

In a way, Roepstorff's work at the Danish Pavilion embodies the spirit of the viral. The pavilion had an uncanny physical and structural resemblance to a virus-like creature. Its boundaries could not be defined precisely, as its sculptural structure reached out well beyond the performance space and the space of the pavilion itself. By freely roaming the space, visitors enacted and strengthened the connections between its parts. The installation was transdisciplinary: part sculpture and part architecture, it combined performative and interactive moments, full-on scripted theatre, and light spectacle. The installation powerfully addressed the fear of the unknown: the unknown as something that is not yet known; as something that is feared because it cannot—yet, or ever—be controlled; as something that is so entangled with the world that it can hardly be fully comprehended; and as something that one single discipline, or method, or technology cannot grasp in its complexity, unless several disciplines, methods, or technologies join forces. Viruses have an intimate relationship with the unknown precisely because of the above qualities. With their surprising trajectories and articulations, viruses are a symbol of today's struggle to contain complex phenomena.

This book is not only about viruses. It interrogates the viral in its diverse articulations and through different disciplinary practices. It's about the narratives and the cultural impact that viruses generate when they interact with human and non-human bodies, media, and networks. It is about how these narratives and impacts can circulate with such ease and how they may intersect, how they are assimilated and re-purposed, and how they are approached creatively or turned into creative objects of their own. I interpret the arts as crucial research contributor to the study of viral phenomena and to the comprehension of the viral. Generally, the different determining aspects of viruses are examined separately, with some being prioritized over others. However, artists and collectives who have engaged with viral phenomena and the viral have demonstrated an extraordinary ability to convey the conceptual significance of the viral by using the instruments of science and by communicating scientific and non-scientific, material and emotional content comprehensively, rather than through the lens of one specific discipline.

For instance, the installation at the Danish Pavilion reveals how artistic expression can flesh out the structural and (material) behavioral aspects of a viral phenomenon, communicate its pervasiveness and cross-disciplinary reach, and evoke its emotional and affective significance. By formulating approaches that are not necessarily tied to discipline-specific definitions, but are multifaceted and interdisciplinary, art manifests a potential to bridge disciplinary realms and reveal their connectedness. Artistic work focusing on viruses and the viral suggests new ways to grasp the elusive nature of viruses. The arts become catalysts, easing the connection between different scientific knowledge and socio-cultural responses. In a technoscientific world intent on measuring, predicting, and controlling everything with minute accuracy, the arts reassert the role of the affective and the provisional in the reading of viral phenomena. Not only are the arts able to reveal aspects about viruses that cannot be unveiled through more traditional approaches, they are also introducing new ways to rethink them.

I started researching the significance of viruses and their peculiar qualities several years ago when the sudden rise of SARS and the dissemination of computer viruses with attractive names in the pre-social media era made the relationship between information and biology remarkably obvious. This led me to explore the kinship, both metaphorical and material, of computer and biological viruses. While using these artificially drawn (yet conventionally understood) categories was helpful to flesh out the ability of viruses to span technical and metaphorical territories, it only partially revealed the unexpected circulation of their qualities, their cross-pollination, and their affective and material impact across techno/scientific and human networks.

I became fascinated by two phenomena: first, the way in which some features that are typically ascribed to viruses have been appropriated, both symbolically and materially, intentionally or subconsciously, by creative individuals or business enterprises. This is the case of viral marketing campaigns, viral videos, or viral tactics, the latter as forms of activism. Second, I was taken by how artistic expression and research, whether exploring viruses explicitly or using their behavior and morphology as metaphors and models for something else, had the ability to provide new insights regarding the tangible and visual appearance of viruses, their behavior, the significance of pandemics and cyberthreats, and the emotional responses they generate.

The binary approach juxtaposing information and biology that I had initially embraced did not capture the complexity of viral phenomena and their unforeseeable proliferation. Furthermore, it did not show how this complexity translated into other virally behaving phenomena that deliberately exploited viral qualities in interdisciplinary ways. Finally, it did not help me to explore viruses as extraordinarily wholesome entities inevitably connected to their surroundings and to other organisms. I found that the arts, by virtue of their ability to cross disciplinary boundaries, and their creative and unconventional use of science and technology, were able to illuminate viral occurrences across different areas of study, and to connect different branches of scientific research, popular culture, and the public understanding of viral phenomena.

In introducing these creative and interdisciplinary projects, my goal in this book is not to propose new methods to break down viral complexity, but to find ways to seize, to get a sense of, the ways that viruses exist not as individual and well-rounded beings, but as relational and dynamic vital forces intimately entangled with their surrounding environment, and with their hosts. My goal is to suggest ways to think "beyond the old dichotomy of the living and non-living" or good vs. evil (Brives 2021). These qualities often interfere with the ability to outline the structure of viruses and predict their behavior discretely (even using AI or complicated math modeling schemes) (Brives 2021). They also make their classification and visualization a multilayered and multi-task endeavor (no matter how advanced the technologies and instruments used are).

Viruses are complex phenomena. Like them, many other complex phenomena have been demonstrated to be equally difficult to comprehend. In the same way, a complex phenomenon like climate change cannot be ascribed to one single cause or one type of nature-culture interaction, pandemics, and the viruses that allegedly cause them; malware and the network disruption it triggers cannot be easily fitted into pre-existing (static) categories. Viruses emerge and fade, appearing each time with different magnitude and gravity; they may cause outbreaks or full-on pandemics; they may produce a great deal of anxiety but no biological damage. Computer viruses may disable entire specialized networks (like financial networks or military networks), but leave everything else alone. What is more important, though, is the extent to which the structural idiosyncrasies and the fast spread of viruses, their materializing and disappearing, their iconic significance (in both their informational and biological incarnations) have allowed them to circulate across different domains that are typically considered incompatible. The existence of computer viruses and their stunning similarities with biological viruses, or the rise of viral videos and viral marketing are all very clear examples of such spread (Buiani 2009).

Rather than trying to tame—by measuring and containing—the richness of viruses, I am interested in learning to appreciate them as entangled, borderless, leaky, and unpredictable entities. In fact, I argue that current disciplinary separations and specializations typical of institutional academic tradition are getting in the way of envisioning a more transdisciplinary and therefore more fertile approach to viruses. To transmit a sense of the dynamic configuration of viruses and their exchanges, material and metaphorical, I'd like to suggest that we start assessing the material, metaphorical, phenomenological, and affective nature of viruses in an interdisciplinary fashion: scientific research, social sciences, and the arts should form meaningful alliances.

Once Upon a Virus

In the spring of 2014, an outbreak of the Ebola hemorrhagic fever in West Africa triggered a massive surge of anxiety worldwide. Between March 2014 and January 2016, over 11,000 people in Liberia, Guinea, and Sierra Leone succumbed to the disease (*BBC News* 2016) and many more died in recurring outbreaks in DRC in the following years (*BBC News* 2020). Concerned about the spread of the infection, its high mortality rate, and the apparent difficulties of the affected nations to contain the epidemic, the World Health Organization (WHO) declared the outbreak a "public health emergency of international concern" (WHO 2016). At that point, news media and social media were flooded with dramatic stories and morbid images; concerned nations became screen travelers, and some even decided to close their borders to the air traffic coming from the affected regions.

Critics charged that these measures were politically and culturally fueled, rather than just medically informed. Some saw the decision to isolate countries devastated by a deadly disease as epidemiologically and politically ill-advised (Wolfson 2016). For others, the delay in sending adequate assistance to the countries hit by Ebola was the sad result of pre-existing racism, economic marginalization, and poverty (Phillips 2014). Ultimately, the actions of governments to contain the disease and the media coverage of the Ebola outbreak laid bare its socio-political situatedness, the marginality of its victims (and, conversely, the self-importance of its potential victims in the global North), and the responsibility of media and the public in disseminating and magnifying its dangers (Phillips 2014).

Ebola was not just a medical emergency, or a mere scientific problem. Epidemiology (the science studying the distribution and determinants of pandemics and other diseases in specific populations), virology (the study of the biology of viruses and viral diseases), and other biological and medical sciences (those preoccupied with finding a cure and producing a vaccine) all provided useful information about the disease as disease, explicating it in terms of number of deaths, rate of contagion, survivability, and spread across countries. Similarly, reflections that focused on the politics at play helped unravel the socio-political significance of the pandemic. But physical bodies and international relations were not the only ones to be affected by the virus. Ebola had also taken residency in the mind and imagination of many individuals. While people residing in the countries affected lived in fear and emotional pain (Moran 2017), the rest of the world imagined apocalyptic scenarios, invigorated by social media, and inspired by hundreds of years of literature, disaster and invasion movies, historical accounts and iconography, and racist stereotypes (Duhaime-Ross, Arielle 2014; Roy et al. 2020).

Ebola traveled many different pathways: it spread from body to body, via different news media and social media, causing the fast dissemination of both real and false information. Ebola quickly morphed into a distributed and all-embracing phenomenon, infiltrating bodies, minds, and information networks, including those focusing on medicine, biology, politics, and the arts.

Ebola is only one of the many pandemics affecting populations worldwide. Pandemics have been well-documented and feared for many centuries, producing a vast literature of medical accounts, political commentaries, and personal stories. Ebola was not the last one either. As SARS-CoV-2 spread across the world courtesy of global travel, international and unchecked trade, deforestation, urban density, and other causes still under investigation, the specter of previous pandemics loomed, bringing back many déjà vu, analogies, metaphors, and socio-cultural conflicts.

Computer viruses were added to the list of viral phenomena in the early 1980s. Their association with biological viruses is both due to claims of material analogies between their functionality and structure, as well as to crucial historical coincidences consolidating such claims. In 1983, while documenting a seminar, computer scientist Fred Cohen formulated the working definition of "a major security problem called virus" (Cohen 1987, 4.; see also Cohen's article "Computer Viruses, Theory and Experiments" published in 1987). His dissertation titled "Computer Viruses" is considered the first comprehensive report about computer malware (Parikka 2007). Cohen did not hesitate to name these bits of code proliferating across various computers connected to form a network *viruses,* proceeding to systemically describe them as if they were digital versions of human epidemics. Computer viruses, he argued, are "programs that can 'infect' other programs by modifying them to include a possibly evolved version of themselves" (Cohen 1994, 2).

For Cohen, computer and biological viruses had material affinity because the technical ability of computer viruses to infect and reproduce thanks to the assistance of a host mirrored similar abilities held by biological viruses. The two also had a metaphorical connection, as computer code, like DNA in biology, could be interpreted as the principal building block of (informational) life. Cohen preferred to use a "working definition" (an open definition devoid of any specific technical detail) of viruses, rather than a technical one. Not only did the absence of specificity implicitly authorize Cohen to extend the term virus to other coded agents with similar behavioral patterns, it also contributed to fuel the well-known collective imaginary that draws comparisons between and unifies all types of viruses.

The existence of computer viruses and other potentially malicious code had been known to programmers since the 1970s and had been tested within relatively controlled environments (Dewdney 1985). Computer viruses were also popular in dystopian and cyberpunk literature—the elective disruptive weapons of skilled hackers and cyberheroes. Cohen's comprehensive analysis is the first that explicitly addresses the potential damage viruses could cause, once released into a worldwide network. Since then, the term virus has exceeded its original definition and is used to refer to other types of *malware.* Malware is the term encompassing computer viruses and many other forms of malicious software, such as computer worms, ransomware, spyware, adware, Trojan horses, keyloggers, rootkits, and bootkits. While these forms of malware are technically not computer viruses, they are easily equated to them, because of their malicious intentions (stealing data, or corrupting operating systems). As it will become clear in the next chapters, the iconography, the metaphors, and the language used to describe computer and biological viruses often converge, locked in a seductive and deceptive dance, thanks in part to the original definition provided by Cohen, and serendipitous events such as the rise of the AIDS pandemic, the rise of network computing of the mid-1980s, and the obvious appearance of the first documented cases of disruptive software (Ross 1991). Their importance was noted by the military-industrial complex since computer viruses could pose a threat to security systems and adversely affect entire industries. Just as the Ebola had commanded massive media and popular attention, computer viruses took center stage in talks about network culture and popular culture.

The widespread use—and abuse—of the attribute *viral* is indicative of the propensity to arbitrarily conflate a whole variety of entities and experiences, as if they could be classified under the same conceptual umbrella. The term viral is used to label a set of features and behaviors (both material and conceptual) proper to computer and biological viruses. However, in common parlance these descriptors have been extended to refer to entities and behaviors beyond both the boundaries delimiting viruses as self-contained objects (as strings of code and as bundle of genetic material) and the restricted disciplinary and dimensional realms of the biological and the informational.

That this has happened is perhaps unsurprising, given that computer malware was almost from the beginning discussed using the language used to refer to biological viruses. The linkage in this case seemed natural. The similarities between what we call biological viruses, sources of infectious diseases, and computer viruses in their incarnation as malware, are uncanny and have been explored in many occasions in scholarly texts and in creative work. Specifically, the immaterial makeup and the functioning of computer viruses and worms have been compared to the submicroscopic size and the elusive nature of biological viruses (by some defined as "undead"), and the distributed and often unforeseeable ways they propagate.

The spread of computer viruses through intricately linked information networks can be easily seen as sharing the same patterns of behavior of biological viruses that produce epidemics. File sharing and density of communications across networks cause computer viruses to spread in a way that reminds us of contagions among human populations. The busier the network, the faster the contagion. Computer viruses are then said to be infectious, just like their biological peers.

In many accounts, computer viruses embody fears of data loss and impersonate the idea of the machine gone out of control. According to Galloway and Thacker, this idea of out-of-control machines is generated from a clash between the effective materiality, or the sovereignty of malware and an assumed design that the network ought to follow, or a structure it is supposed to preserve. The way viruses behave, and their inherent and material features, are in conflict with the attempt to control, predict, and dominate them (Galloway and Thacker 2007). In a society depending on computing and online connectivity aimed at fulfilling certain well-planned tasks, malware could pose a very real threat to productivity and daily routines, and therefore to people's livelihood. A range of activities, including work and social life, government services, and the network infrastructure to guarantee our physical and psychical well-being, could be affected.

The term viral is then used to denote one or all the features that in a general way, or in a popular way, characterize both informational and biological viral agents. For instance, it can describe the exceptionally pervasive dissemination of Ebola as both a biological agent and as a series of news bytes. This "spillover" effect has taken the most evident form during the 2020 coronavirus pandemic: the virus—possibly—jumped from a species to another and invaded the realm of information, as the comparisons between the spread of the real virus and what the World Health Organization calls *infodemics*—the intentional or inadvertent circulation of false and inaccurate information—demonstrate (Ball and Maxmen 2020; Boot 2020; Caulfield 2020; Dominguez 2020; WHO—Health Topics 2020).

I am not interested in developing a symmetrical comparison between computer and biological viruses. Examining the intersection between computer and biological viruses is indeed important, but not because it shows how many items they share in real life, but because this connection is the best possible example of how narratives travel across the biological and the informational through analogies and metaphors, and how easily certain ideas about viruses are appropriated and applied elsewhere. Furthermore, it shows how the traffic between information and biology (Haraway 1988; Schneider 2012) has not only enabled the circulation of common narratives that all viruses share, but it has also validated the application of terms and methodologies across biology and computer science.

As viruses spread thanks to the viral, generating news and fear of contagion, and transforming into other objects and phenomena, their trajectory and structure appear to be dynamically open-ended (as opposed to self-contained and fixed). Dealing with such lack of closure and transience may cause a lingering sense of discomfort and can have paralyzing effects. However, the same discomfort can be also surprisingly productive, thus triggering new investigations, experimentation, and openness to venture into uncharted territories. Examining the creative and artistic appropriation and independent explorations of viruses is helpful to understand the ways individuals familiarize themselves with viruses, and how they may develop new strategies to cope with such aleatory, confusing, and volatile phenomena. In their use of the viral, artists show us potential new strategies for dealing with other complex and/or unknown phenomena.

Going Interdisciplinary

The first major deadly pandemic in one hundred years raged across the world in 2020–22. Last time a pandemic event had reached such magnitude, 50 million people had died between 1918 and 1920 ("1918 Pandemic (H1N1 Virus) | Pandemic Influenza (Flu) | CDC" 2020). SARS-CoV-2 seems to have taken everybody by surprise. In fact, SARS-CoV-2 emerged suddenly, but we cannot say that scientists didn't see it coming. As it is the case of many other zoonotic diseases, SARS-CoV-2 could be the result of a spillover.

The Spanish flu, before it, is known to have an avian origin. Scientists supporting this hypothesis tell us that a spillover is a phenomenon we have become accustomed to seeing more frequently thanks to the combination of industrial farming and deforestation, extension of urban settlements, and increased mobility of humans and animals (Quanmen 2013; Shah 2017). Epidemics are often blamed on the traffic of wild animals at wet markets and the consumption of bush meat, but as Ed Yong reminds us, quoting ecologist Colin Carlton, "the biggest factors behind spillovers are land-use change and climate change" (Yong 2020a). SARS-CoV-2 circulated virtually undisturbed for months, despite early records of a mysterious anomalous pneumonia suddenly raising concerns among the medical community (Andersen et al. 2020; Wang 2020; WHO 2020).

While the causes of pandemics are known, predicting their emergence with precision is unlikely possible. The problem is not that we don't have technologies to monitor and track what triggers pandemics, but that too many variables converge to cause them. For years, the World Health Organization (WHO), the Centers for Disease Control and Prevention (CDC), and other international health organizations have been monitoring emerging infectious diseases and have warned about their pandemic potentials. However, many predictions did not become a reality. In fact, they were based on small sets of data or historical data with no guarantee of accuracy. For instance, during the 2020 pandemic, a variety of mathematical models was enlisted to predict the trajectory and behavior of the pandemic. Because of lack of data, because of unexpected factors affecting the outcome of the model, or simply because of human error, these models were not always able to make accurate predictions (Cepelewicz 2021; Murty 2021). Importantly, pandemics affect different countries in different ways: cultural practices, socioeconomic configuration, industrial and demographic geographies, environmental conditions, density of population, family habits, policy decisions, and many more factors may affect or change the course of a pandemic.

Similar difficulties are likely caused by the variables and the unknowns contributing to malware and computer security breaches. As soon as a new malware is detected, security firms rush to create security updates that may or may not protect the user from cyberattacks. In part, this may depend on the user's security settings, their computer literacy, or their behavior. In this case too, failure to predict or to protect the host computer is not caused by technological error, but by the interplay of the many variables characterizing network environments, including users' computer literacy or their risky online behavior.

Blaming absence or inadequacy of technological and scientific tools for the failure to predict outbreaks or to protect oneself from cyberattacks is a simplistic course of action. Yet, a disproportionate amount of trust is placed on technologies that monitor, measure, see, and predict epidemics and cybersecurity threats. Humans display a deep-seated desire to control things and, even more importantly, concepts. Inevitably, when this desire meets with failure, it produces frustration. Attempts to explore increasingly complex phenomena and to tame the unknown can be accompanied by fear, which often results in a reluctance to deal with such unknown or, conversely, to venture into uncharted territories (Virilio 2000). The same uncomfortable sense of frustration accompanies perceived instrumental failure, that is, when one realizes that a particular mode of knowledge-seeking that finds it comforting to deal with discrete data and precise measurements becomes outdated or does no longer apply to achieve a certain knowledge or to solve a specific problem (Robins and Webster 1999).

Rather than new technologies, interdisciplinary approaches are needed not only to provide a multifaceted and diversified—not complete or comprehensive—view on complicated phenomena, but also to help comprehend the uncertainty and anxiety that these phenomena produce. Thus, the question to be asked is not with which technology, discipline, or method should we map, visualize, control, delimit, or fully understand this or that disease, this or that outbreak? But can we find a discourse, behavior, or overall methodology that will help us come to terms with viruses and other viral phenomena?

Coming to terms doesn't mean to passively accept the cyclical and/or unexpected occurring of viral episodes; it doesn't mean that we should just wait for the flu or the next pandemic to come without doing anything; it doesn't mean that we shouldn't upgrade our antivirus software regularly. Rather, it means that we should find ways to cope with the uncertainty that these phenomena cause by addressing them differently; that we should become aware of their elusive behavior and nature, their overall complexity, by observing them from different angles, or by assessing their impact both on the human and the non-human.

Contemporary conventional Western thought[1] appears to have hit a particular socio-cultural, political, and epistemological conjuncture: extensive research has been produced to examine the structure and transformations of viruses and pandemics, the forces and events that cause climate change, and the political and economic unrests that lead to terror and its wars. However, it is not the danger caused by a pandemic or a cyberattack per se that terrifies the most, but the perception that they cannot be fully controlled, even when specialized tools are used to predict their outcomes and powerful measures are taken against them. There is an increasing awareness of the difficulty in

[1]As a non-native English-speaking scholar born in Southern Europe, I like to refer to Western thought or "the West" as per Edward Said and Stuart Hall definition as an "archive or a family of ideas" and "a unifying set of values proven in various ways to be effective" (Hall 2018). According to Linda Tuhiwai Smith " ... what counts as Western research draws from an 'archive' of knowledge and systems, rules and values which stretch beyond the boundaries of Western science to the system now referred to as the West" (Tuhiwai Smith 2021).

predicting and controlling their occurring, as creating more monitoring and measuring technologies, or mathematical models is often not sufficient to resolve them. This situation poses a challenge to the way hyper-specialized research is structured today.

This issue then begs the question: is it more important to know more, hoping that this additional knowledge will help us decipher a phenomenon fully and anticipate its outcomes, or would it make better sense to know how to cope with, be prepared to embrace the uncertainty that pandemics and malware generate? How crucial is it to control these entities? And can we control them? And for the benefit of whom? Can we see beyond human exceptionalism, the human tendency to think of ourselves at the center of the world?

The structure of this book shows how, to capture the rich articulation of viruses, it is imperative to use a multivocal, transdisciplinary lens. Each of its sections starts with specific approaches and methods to study viruses and viral phenomena, showing that these approaches are already the result of a convergence of different disciplines. Virology and epidemiology engage in frequent methodology exchanges involving medical and biological sciences, mathematics, and information technology. These intersections are not only needed because of the complex nature of the phenomena studied, but also because the proliferation of the viral across biology and information calls for a crosspollination between methods used to fight diseases and methods employed to limit cyberattacks.

Chapter 1 to 6 examine a set of methods typically used to study viruses and their informational kin in their material structure, such as taxonomy and naming, microscopy and molecular modeling, and through their dynamic distribution, through mapping and mathematical modeling. Chapter 7 and 8 observes how viruses “go viral” when their qualities are opportunistically appropriated or embraced outside of their original context. Throughout each chapter, it becomes clear that individual disciplinary approaches are not tenable in the study and the comprehension of viruses. In order to achieve a richer understanding, alliances between different research groups are necessary; an ecology of technologies will have to participate in dissecting, classifying, and rendering viruses; methods and individuals must be placed in dialogue with one another. I acknowledge the generative relations that these alliances form in reaching better, sharper, more precise knowledge of these invisible genetic bundles and strings of code. However, in this book, I am not interested in merely identifying the common qualities of viruses, or in finding new ways to dissect them, or in classifying them as analog or digital, mental or corporeal. Instead, I invite the reader to consider the whimsical and complicated nature of viruses and their relations within and as part of the contexts they interact with, their integration and intertwining with the world that surrounds them, the communities they affect, be they the biological, informational, or metaphorical world.

Specialized studies that strictly rely on one body of knowledge are not (or not necessarily) sufficient to understand the spread of a pathogen that depends on individuals' mobility as well as on socially dense exchanges to thrive. As Tom Koch explains in his *Disease Maps* (2011), different approaches and the study of different variables are needed to start understanding an epidemic. The identification by John Snow of the London Broad Street outbreak of cholera in 1866 included a series of actions that at the time were considered radical: they included not only laying down a disease on a map but also conducting research on the ground. This interdisciplinary approach inaugurated a new era in the study of epidemiology and marked the beginning of the study of infectious diseases as biosocial occurrences rather than as self-sustained and independent events, that is, as incidents that not only affected, but also actively involved entire communities[2].

Many years later, in 2006, a few years before Ebola, and a few years after the SARS and the AIDS pandemics, a joint study by physicists Dirk Brockman and Dirk Helbing, respectively from the Max Planck Institute for Dynamics and Self-Organization in Göttingen University and the University of California Santa Barbara, proposed a new mathematical theory to map the spread of infectious diseases (Brockman 2007). Rather than basing their research on the transmission of pathogens from body to body, and from country to country, the team built a mathematical model based on the geographic circulation of millions of one-dollar bills, tracked through a website titled "wheresgeorge.com" (Rocketboom n.d; "Where's George? Currency Tracking Project" 2016). It was thanks to this everyday item, to a non-scientific and non-medical device—a common banknote—that the two scientists performed their predictions. The study led to the discovery of universal scaling laws in human mobility, and the forecast of spreading routes of the 2009 flu epidemic in the United States. The study was possible because the researchers chose to look at habitual, everyday mobility and exchange patterns, patterns that would determine the route that a potential infectious disease would likely take.

The Role of the Arts

With all viruses relying on networks—digital and physical, human and non-human—to proliferate, determining where they will land next is a challenging business. In part, this is because of their complicated structure and extensive dissemination. However, research is also often caught in discipline-driven

[2]While populations living in urban areas had noticed that certain incidences tended to affect specific neighborhoods, Fine et al. note: "Whether or not John Snow should be regarded as the father of epidemiology is open to debate, because some of his predecessors such as William Farr might also be credited with such a distinction. However, Snow was unquestionably an essential link in the causal chain that led epidemiology to what it is now. His ingenuity in placing cholera cases on a geographical grid, and in comparing cholera incidence according to sources of household water supply, constituted groundbreaking innovations in the development of the epidemiological approach" (Fine et Al. 2013).

structures meant to produce discrete data. In addition, the fields of information technology and biology often assume that advanced technologies produce better data when they produce more of them. Furthermore, failures to capture the complexity of viruses, their movements, and their impact are also the product of epistemological shortcomings to grasp the invisible and the abstract. Viruses and the contexts they are attached to often feel like elusive objects exactly because of these shortcomings. In fact, tangible and measurable characteristics are important, but they go hand in hand with less verifiable—invisible or undetectable—qualities. Neither viruses nor the context they inhabit can be precisely captured or measured; nor can the public perception of viruses and pandemics be completely defined or articulated, as no individual is affected by or experiences them in the same way.

Here is where I believe lies the crucial role of interdisciplinary approaches and artistic interpretations. The arts invite us to think past disciplinary constraints and to conceive of viruses as situated in and entangled with their surroundings, be they human or non-human, by displaying the rich ecologies formed by viruses and viral phenomena and by suggesting new approaches and ways to capture their aleatory, elusive, unspeakable, and puzzling nature. In this book, I emphasize the importance of coupling critical and technical reflections on viruses and viral processes with artworks that reflect on, engage with, and embrace their qualities and behavior.

Artists have been particularly interested in exploring the many vectors that constitute viral phenomena and in questioning the current propensity to fit viruses into predetermined grids and well-contoured categories: partly as a challenge to the material and conceptual difficulties currently preventing the sciences from defining viruses, partly to garner publicity by capitalizing on the infamous popularity of the biological and informational incarnations of viruses, and partly as a genuine desire to find new ways to understand them, artists and creative individuals have represented, reproduced, and explained how viruses look, how they spread, and how they communicate and affect both our bodies and information and technical networks.

Importantly, many of the artists engaging with this topic tend to operate outside of specific disciplinary areas and often mix different media and approaches: they are either temporary guests of a lab or amateur scientists, and typically create artworks that not always comply with specific scientific protocols. Sometimes, they have a science background but do not work in scientific institutions. Their existence outside of a lab or outside of an institutional situation has provided them with a great deal of freedom and the ability to venture beyond the disciplinary boundaries established by the institution. As artists gradually learn about the scientific instruments used to examine viruses, study the effects of viruses, speak to experts, and read media coverage about epidemic outbreaks, they locate the process of engagement with viruses and viral phenomena at the core of their artistic practice. This process-based exploration is radically different from the outcome-driven objectives of scientific and technological research, where the goal is to find a solution, a device, or a statistical model (in other words, a discrete entity) able to summarize a phenomenon once and for all.

This type of work is seldom recognized as having scientific significance. It also tends to escape genre classification or identification with a specific and/or recognizable art practice. But it is thanks to this very (liminal and privileged) position at the intersection of distinct areas (the sciences, the arts, and popular culture) that artists can explore topics that professional scientists are not interested in or cannot investigate on their own, and display views and hypotheses that are not institutionally-approved.

This openness also interprets viruses as relational objects determined by, and through the ecologies in which they are immersed and which they form (Barad 2007). The contribution of the arts is crucial in making such complexity tangible and in making public those qualities of the viral that had been ignored or cannot be considered for further exploration. These include the non-measurable elements normally excluded from scientific analysis, such as the affective and biosocial aspects of viruses originating from personal and collective reactions to pandemics, and the ambiguous blurring of the boundaries between science fiction and popular science, which both reflect and affect the way science and technology deal with viruses.

Blending Visions

In this book, I wish to blend traditional methods and research on viruses with the way in which artists, creative individuals, and scientists—working in a biological and informational context, in and outside the laboratory—have used, re-elaborated, bypassed, and re-imagined disciplinary constraints and obligations, formalities, and normative processes of inclusion and exclusion on and around viruses. Critical discourse analysis and media/visual analysis assisted me in establishing a dialogue between disciplines such as STS and Media Studies and scholarship within the social sciences that often lie separate despite sharing a range of topics and interests. These same frameworks also helped me draw frequent connections between computer science and biology.

Each chapter draws on different approaches used by the sciences to study viruses and their dissemination: this includes isolating, naming, and classifying viruses (Chapters 1 and 2), visualizing and imaging viruses (Chapter 3), mapping and modeling to predict their trajectory, in order to protect us from viral threats (Chapters 4 and 5), and establishing narratives to raise awareness of their danger, facing and embracing them (Chapters 6 and 7). Looming over each chapter is the big shadow cast by the virus that we (or at least scientists) have been anticipating for many decades and now we all experienced in all its marvelous, disruptive, and dramatic power.

SARS-CoV-2 descended upon the world like a meteor, causing death and long-term suffering in many individuals it encountered, economic collapse of entire sectors, social and political turmoil. But pandemics are not able to create such chaos on their own: David Barnes and Françoise Baylis define them as "inequality accelerators" (UPenn Arts & Sciences: David Barnes 2020; Herzberg 2020). Never has this pandemic made it so clear. This book contained already in its previous versions plenty of examples demonstrating how pandemics are not creating but exacerbating already existing inequalities and other cracks in the socioeconomic system. However, the current situation, and the events that ensued, made it absolutely necessary to incorporate a more thorough analysis responding to the coronavirus pandemic of 2020.

Viruses are immersed in a rich environment made of proteins, DNA strands, cell tissue, and in a complex and intricate network of connections with other agents and data. In fact, without this richness surrounding them, they would not survive. Yet, if viruses are always found in "good company," then why do science and popular culture alike imagine them in isolation, as if they were self-contained entities with a powerful agency? Why do we name, classify, and isolate viruses the way we do? And do we have a choice? Chapter 1 asks these questions: despite growing awareness of the entangled and relational nature of viruses, textbooks and visual illustrations do not reflect such findings. On the one hand, statements about the nature of viruses describe them as diffused, interconnected, and often symbiotic. The same ideas are accompanied by the persistence of terminology and principles of classification that contradict such description, because they insert the virus into a structural and genetic container and ascribe to viruses a disproportionate amount of agency. The classic images of viruses isolated and emerging from a void background illustrate this conflict visually, while attempts at changing this visual paradigm, such as in the case of the molecular landscapes by David Goodsell, are still rare. Its origin pertains to the complicated and ephemeral nature of viruses as well as to the apparatus of knowledge that has dominated science for many years before it was possible to seize viruses with more clarity.

Chapter 2 focuses on how the relationship between information technology and biology is reflected in the manipulation, digitization, and simplification leading to the visualization of viruses. We rarely speculate about what processes have led to the illustration of a virus. This process is the product of an interesting circular exchange involving information and biology. This exchange originates from the drive to control molecular material as information. Shannon and Weaver's mathematical theory of communication and the genomic turn taught us to think of the biological and the informational as realms whose principles can be compared and to a certain extent made interchangeable. In fact, be they genes, or bits of code, both digital machines and biological beings are made to be dissected and measured through discrete packets. As models and renditions make viruses more legible, the colors and shades, the geometric forms they display, and other qualities employed in these renditions appear to undermine the reality they represent. For instance, the tendency to represent viruses as isolated entities, and the fact that informational and biological viruses are often encased in well-defined visual structures, testify to the persistence of generalizations and common beliefs regarding the nature and effects of viruses. The recurrence of predetermined and discrete characteristics in descriptions and representation of viruses expresses a desire to produce clarity without violating the rules and obligations that govern scientific and technical knowledge.

In Chapter 2, I consider two radically different images, respectively the work of interdisciplinary artist and sculptor Luke Jerram and designer and programmer Alex Dragulescu. The first one is a glass sculpture of the molecular model of the Avian Flu (also known as H5N1). The second one is a digital illustration of MyDoom, a computer worm mainly affecting Windows operating systems. The two works demonstrate the extent to which methods and conventional forms of representation not only are preserved in radically different renditions of viruses, but they are also exchanged across the realms of biology (Jerram) and information (Dragulescu). In both cases, generalizations are used out of necessity and as a convenient move to either construct a material, tangible item where there is originally none (as in Dragulescu), or to highlight the way in which many elements composing viruses are manipulated and constructed to direct the viewer's perception of a certain entity (Jerram).

While Chapter 2 shows how the difficulties involved in describing, defining, and visualizing viruses are both ontological (due to their nature) and epistemological (due to their qualities as cultural constructs and as products of a convergence of vectors) in nature, Chapter 3 zooms in on the popular, yet relatively recent art of visualization. Here, understanding the role of visualization as a process and not as a static product, and examining the way in which this process has been re-interpreted by artists takes center stage. As artist Tagny Duff argues, viruses are simultaneously "entity" and "movement," "living" and "undead," "material" and "dynamic" (Duff 2009).

The now iconic red and white model of SARS-CoV2 created in February 2020 by Alissa Eckert and Dan Higgins for the Centers for Disease Control and Prevention (CDC) and Veronica Falconieri Hays' 3D model of the virus produced for the July 2020 special issue of *Scientific American* are well-documented best practice in visualization, showing how the shapes and components of the coronavirus have been partly inferred from existing models (the first SARS virus being an important start), selected from different research labs, or arbitrary determined (the choice to display or not display a stem in the spikes, the choice of colors).

With their composite, performative pieces, artists Caitlin Berrigan (Berrigan 2009) and Tagny Duff (Duff et al. 2011) demonstrate how viruses exceed the visual and structural constraints that science and conventional aesthetics have assigned to them. The two artists translate scientific facts and personal information into different media formats, the former through a series of chocolate sculptures faithfully shaped after the molecular model of hepatitis C retrieved from the Worldwide Protein Data Bank; the second, by indicating the presence of viruses using bio-markers "tattooed" on human and pig tissue. In both cases, viruses are inserted in a series of executions—rather than one sole image—that evoke the physical presence of the virus and its effects, its popular conception, and its existence and visual manifestation through technological instruments and laboratory processes.

In Chapter 4, I explore another function of imaging: the technologies and techniques used to examine and process viruses tend to create a physical and perceived distance between the viewer and the object analyzed. This distance is certainly produced by practical needs, but also reflects a propensity to simultaneously control and protect (or protect themselves against) the object. In this chapter, I turn my attention to how seeing as a crucial form of knowledge fulfills a cultural need for taming and protecting oneself from the unknown. With the unknown being associated historically with fear, and with darkness as, itself, a generator of fear, seeing becomes a way to neutralize fear; technologies as tools to prepare, filter, manipulate, and present viruses create a safe distance between the observer and the object and become a protection not only against the unknown but also against the threat caused by the virus. The work by transdisciplinary artist Laura Splan in her 2004 SARS Doilies and her animations of the protein spikes of SARS-CoV2 reproduce the virus by using the familiar craft of lace and by treating the visualization software as a medium to manipulate the proteins of the virus aesthetically. Both her works show the mediated nature of biomolecular visualization as well as its protective function. Visualizations of computer viruses are notably rare and generally considered less crucial to the understanding and study of malware. However, the one being disseminated today may help better elucidate the notion of distancing as control, defense, and protection.

While the previous chapters mainly examine the relational nature and inner structure of viruses, Chapters 5 and 6 delve into their epidemiological distribution, that is, the way they spread across human and non-human networks and geographical areas, their behavioral patterns, and the way they can be predicted and contained. In Chapter 5, I focus on two important technical tools of epidemiological research: epidemiological maps and mathematical models. The display and communication of viral data by means of epidemiological maps and models lead to the creation, the strengthening, or the challenging of narratives shaping infections and outbreaks. My emphasis is not on the technical intricacy or on the accuracy of epidemiological maps and projections, but on the stories they produce and communicate.

In examining the maps and mathematical projections about the outbreaks occurring in computer networks and in the real world, I reflect on the collective narratives they generate. What do they prioritize and what population do they speak to? What do they miss? How can artistic work function as a reminder of these absences? And how can it address these absences?

In this chapter, I argue that these narratives, as helpful and as compelling as they are, often dismiss the impact of infectious diseases on non-hegemonic and minority groups and their histories, and I call for a more situated kind of epidemiological work that enabled this portion of the population not only to be better represented, but also to be heard.

The recent interdisciplinary project Visualizing the Virus led by Sria Chatterjee presents a kaleidoscopic collection of the many ways SARS-Cov2 (the virus) is being visualized—both by science and by different communities. In addition, it attempts to map and expose the inequalities that the virus has suddenly made visible with its passing, by naming the hierarchies and the exclusions that COVID-19 (the disease) has produced during its passage. These are all aspects that traditional maps and models are currently unable to underscore. Similarly, Anna Dumitriu's ex voto installation features stories of individuals who had personal encounters with the disease. The uniqueness of these stories reveals a set of experiences that epidemiological data could not seize by design, and that members of the medical profession unfortunately are in many cases forced to ignore, because they are usually deemed anecdotal. While Dumitriu illuminates personal stories, Ruth Cuthand's series Trading and Surviving reappropriates recurring symbols of the pandemic to create an alternative narrative that this time gives voice to her ancestors.

Epidemiological maps and models contribute to outbreak narratives, since they use design to create infectious stories that may raise awareness about an impending—medical or networked—threat or may direct government decision making and policy changes. In Chapter 6, I move my attention to examining how outbreak narratives modulate different degrees of affect. The symbols and objects, metaphors and tropes, the refrains and the sound bites used in the perpetuation of outbreak narratives produce very different emotional responses: these may depend on personal and collective experiences of a disease; they may display a range of emotions from fear to anxiety to a sense of inevitability; they may cause individuals to freeze or to dare venturing into the unknown.

Elaine Whittaker's installations explore how objects and symbols of infectious disease generate different affective responses lingering in both scientific accounts and popular culture/cinematic narratives, and simultaneously materializing as collective historical experiences and personal stories. The series of science fiction performances by Micha Cárdenas and Elle Mehrmand, Virus.Circus, re-imagine the collective and personal perceptions of viral occurrences, through the choices that people make in the face of the risks viruses pose, treating them as opportunities for dialogue and for creative disruption rather than just as insurmountable and paralyzing obstacles.

Chapter 7 pushes the notion of the viral further: to what degree, how, and in what circumstances is/can the viral be embraced, either as part of an ongoing artistic work or as part of the journey of a group or an individual. How can we better cope with and embrace the viral? What if, instead of fearing the worst, we decide to acknowledge the unpredictable outcome of viruses? What if we learn how to cope with the capricious nature of these phenomena? This chapter invites us to search for a different modus vivendi able to coexist with those partial, complex, and multifaceted phenomena that cannot be captured or understood in their totality, nor perceived in universal ways.

This chapter leads us to examine computer science search for the "good virus" and medicine's re-discovery of the powerful qualities of bacteriophage, an unlikely ally in the fight against antibiotic resistance. The artists and collectives I examine in this chapter show an open-minded approach to the potentials of the viral, to the multiplicity of relations contributing to its formation and circulation, and to the aleatory features of biological viruses and their computer counterparts. One important aspect emerges from these interventions: openness toward viruses, whether informational or biological, was dictated by the curiosity to find out how far the viral would go, what opportunities it would bring about, and what new aesthetics it would generate. The dangerous aspects of viruses were not just used to cause clamor, but also to draw attention to specific and important issues that would otherwise lie hidden. This is not to downplay the disruptive power of viruses or the suffering of those in most vulnerable positions. In acknowledging such sufferings, it is important to also give voice to alternative strategies to exercise, embrace, or comprehend viruses. This is the case of *La Cura* by Salvatore Iaconesi and Oriana Persico, whose drive to go viral was not just an attempt to crowdsource a cure for cancer, but also, and more importantly, to create a stronger community in the name of care.

The work of PeiYing Lin offers a series of speculative performances focused on how to live with viruses, and how to welcome their ubiquitous presence into everyday activities. To various degrees, and driven by radically different goals, Joseph Nechvatal and the duo 0100101110101101.org, known today as Eva and Franco Mattes, showed us the ability of the viral to cross domains and media, and embraced its open-ended outcomes and its resistance to human control. These artists seem to be less interested in exploiting the qualities of viruses for personal or financial gain and more interested in exploring their merging and entanglement with the surrounding environment and the nearby culture, their becoming something different at each of these encounters, and their ability to transform these environments and cultures. Nechvatal's use of the viractual in his artistic practice is meant to reveal "the power of digitization while being culturally aware of the values of monumentality and permanency" (Nechvatal 2002).

1

Virological Ambiguities

The Lone Wanderer

It emerges from a dark space, with colorful contours and intricate shapes: *hic sunt dracones* the saying goes. The virus is a jewel in a sea of darkness. Polished, colorful, and camera-ready, it appears suspended in time and space, as if it was posing for a commemorative photograph; it looks more like a natural history specimen in a glass showcase than an active agent ready to infect the host.

Figure 1 is an atomic model of the SARS-CoV-2 virion[1], that is, a molecular visualization of the entire virus particle in its non-entangled, non-active state, composed of an outer protein shell called a capsid and an inner core of nucleic acid (Dupré and Guttinger 2016). This is only one of the images created thanks to a collaboration between KAUST (King Abdullah University of Science and Technology), the Research Unit of Computer Graphics at TU Wien (Wien Technical University), and the Scripps Research Institute. The image exists as a standalone high-resolution image that can be downloaded for free and studied. This is one of the many visualizations and illustrations increasingly circulating in news media and popular culture; in magazines and journals.

For now, I will not examine the technical wizardry that led to the creation of this image (this will be the topic of Chapter 3). In this chapter, I want to draw attention to the format and layout of this image. This suspended view is accepted as THE way in which viruses look and should be visualized. The same format appears on the covers of magazines (such as *Scientific American* or *The New Scientist*), academic journals (such as *Science, Nature*, or *The*

[1]The image has been reconstructed thanks to modeling and visualization techniques that take into consideration both microscopy images and simulations and models extracted from the Protein Data Bank. Nguyen et al. claim that this model renders the "full hierarchical structure of living organisms—from atoms to cells."

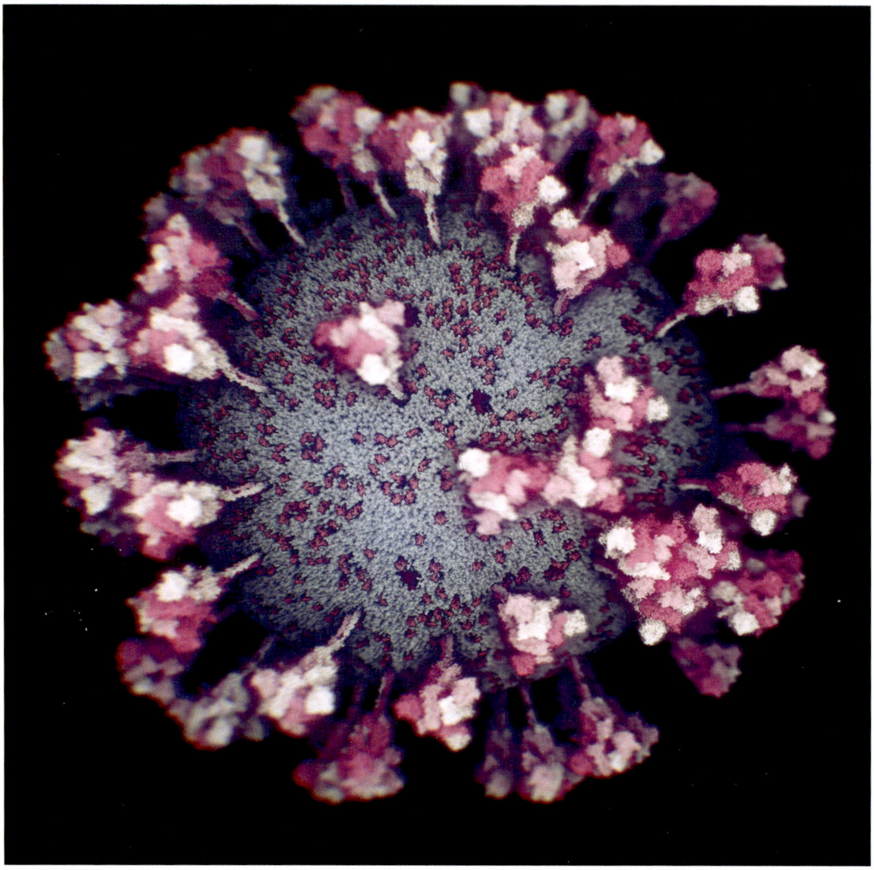

FIGURE 1 *Image of SARS-CoV-2 Atomistic model made by Nanographics GmbH. "Resulting 3D models are based on few 2D microscopy scans and the latest knowledge about the biological entity represented as a set of geometric relationships. Our new technique is based on statistical and rule-based modeling approaches that are rapid to author, fast to construct, and easy to revise" (Nguyen et al. 2020). Work licensed under the Creative Commons Attribution 4.0 International License version 2020-05-17.*

Journal of Medical Virology), and textbooks on virology and epidemiology (both as detailed illustrations and as schematics). But viruses are never alone: they float in a soup filled with different particles: proteins, DNA strands, cell tissue, etc. In fact, without this environmental richness surrounding them, they would not survive (nor would they have any reason to). If this is true, then why is the richness surrounding and interacting with the virus made invisible? If viruses are always found in "good company," in a rich context which includes several organisms, environmental elements, and the host, then why is science and popular culture alike treating them as if they were self-contained entities with a powerful agency? Why do we (mainstream science, art, and popular culture) persist in naming, classifying, and isolating viruses the way we do? And is there any choice?

These questions are at the core of this chapter. Recent findings about viruses are only partially reflected in the way they are taught in schools through the discipline of virology, and how they are included in taxonomic classification. On the one hand, statements about the nature of viruses describe them as entangled, diffused, interconnected, and symbiotic. On the other hand, the same ideas are accompanied by the persistence of terminology and principles of classification that contradict such description, inserting the virus into a structural and genetic container and ascribing to viruses a disproportionate amount of agency. The typical images of viruses isolated and emerging from a void background illustrate this conflict visually. The nature of this series of discrepancies is both ontological and epistemological, as it pertains to the complicated and ephemeral nature of viruses as well as to the apparatus of knowledge that has dominated science for many years before it was possible to seize viruses with more clarity. In addition, it applies to biological viruses as much as it does as to computer viruses. In the latter case, the issue of immateriality, translated as code abstractness, authorizes and even encourages the overlapping between information and biology, inspiring artists and computer scientists to adapt similar iconographic and discursive qualities originally ascribed to their biological relatives to descriptions and illustrations.

Conflicted Nature

Viruses "occupy a unique position in biology" (Van Regenmortel and Fauquet 2000). As entities carrying either DNA or RNA (but not both), they lack the genetic apparatus that would allow them to replicate on their own. This aspect places them in " … a gray area between living and nonliving: they cannot replicate on their own but can do so, in truly living cells and can also affect the behavior of their hosts profoundly" (Villarreal 2005). More precisely, they exist "at the intersection of chemistry and life" (Villarreal 2008); in a hospitable environment, they become active, just as a chemical reaction is triggered by the presence of a specific enzyme or by the proximity to a particularly attractive element. Outside of that environment, they cease to function. Yet, they still qualify as viruses; they must rely on other organisms to survive and be transported. This aspect suggests that viruses do not exist in just one fixed state.

In describing viruses, Villarreal states that previous trends in science have focused on viruses as predominantly disease-carrying entities: this interpretation, he argues, has caused many scientists to overlook the crucial "viral contributions to the history of life on earth" (Villarreal 2008). The problem in part lies in the abundance of the viral population, as current estimates agree that 10^{31} individual viruses and counting exist on this planet, a number too large to even imagine. In part, however, this focus is due to the necessity of virology to prioritize viruses affecting or deadly to human beings and other organisms connected to humans (like cattle and other farm animals, plants, and other organisms deemed useful to the thriving of the human species) (Gorbalenya et al. 2020; Simmonds et al. 2017). In fact, despite the bad reputation, terror, and panic that human and animal pandemics have caused, only a small variety of the trillions of viruses known and unknown today are dangerous. Most are not only innocuous, but also fundamental to promoting natural evolution. Viruses are an unavoidable presence in our oceans, in our food, and in our gut (along with several million bacteria). It is believed that our genome reached today's complexity thanks to viruses (Cobián Güemes et al. 2016; Moelling 2017, 6). Because of the many activities that constitute the viral life cycle, and because of the different states and roles they exist in, Dupré and Guttinger argue that viruses should not be interpreted as stable matter and distinct entities, but as processes (Dupré and Guttinger 2016).

When it comes to the domain of information, computer viruses and malware are often treated in ways that very closely remind us of the treatment of their biological kin. They are identified, and subsequently dealt with, according to the potential damage that they may cause. Because they are classified as fundamentally dangerous, it is easy to forget that they are actually part of a very rich digital environment where agency is mostly distributed: computer viruses, worms, spyware, ransomware, spread across cyberspace's networks and nodes, following trajectories that closely mimic human communications traffic; sometimes their spread appears random and disorienting. Knowing where they will land and what their trajectory will be depends on projections and statistics (Alt 2005). Manifesting behavioral patterns reminiscent of biological outbreaks, malware spreads thanks to busy web traffic, social activities, and frequent business exchanges. Malware appears to follow busy networks, in the same way that biological viruses expand across densely populated areas and intense human circulation (and animal trade), in conjunction with global mobility trends. Malware would not spread, and certainly not at this rate, without today's fast means of communication.

Both biological and computer viruses share one crucial quality: their nature is relational and processual. While they both contain a basic genetic or coded essence, their liveliness is connected with, and dependent on, their host, as well as on the abundance of potential hosts creating the advantageous conditions for their thriving and reproduction. Thus, their boundaries are not completely clear, or they are subject to change at any time. Given recent discoveries about coevolution and coexistence, DNA exchanges, zoonotic transfers, and network studies confirming the dependence of viruses upon complex relations (Cobián Güemes et al. 2016; E. Cohen 2011; Galloway 2007; Hinterberger and Porter 2015; Moelling 2013), the clear separation between the human and the viral based on the traditional way of thinking is becoming increasingly difficult to defend. Although the entangled multi-state nature of viruses is well known to professionals and scientists in the field, it doesn't appear to be acknowledged fully when it comes to naming and classification, and as a consequence, the representation of viruses.

Several scientific accounts have confirmed the crucial role that viruses have played in a variety of evolutionary processes and in the production of oxygen for the survival of carbon-based organisms (Moelling 2013). For instance, Caetano-Anolles and Nasir analyzed the protein folds of over 5,000 organisms and discovered that while "442 protein folds were shared between cells and viruses [only] 66 folds ... were unique to viruses" (Milliken 2015). This discovery suggests that viruses once shared properties with cells and later evolved as separate entities. Caetano-Anolles says that this discovery confirms that viruses are not only crucial to life but that they are also alive. This is an important statement because scientists' view of liveliness in viruses "influences their thinking about the mechanisms of evolution" (Villarreal 2008). Milliken states: "The mere fact of the existence of a universal biology unifying viruses and cells now justifies the construction of a Tree of Life that embraces viruses side by side with cells" (Milliken 2015).

Furthermore, it is a well-known fact that retroviruses tend to remain in the host's system by hiding in their DNA (Ashley et al. 2018; Callier 2018; Cepelewicz 2017). Sometimes, a retrovirus will mix with the genome of an egg or sperm. Embryos will carry a copy of the virus in every single cell—including its own egg or sperm. When viruses stay active, they will still multiply and keep mixing with the host's genome: they will literally be inherited from parents to children to grandchildren. This process, Zimmer explains, generates a "huge amount of viral DNA in the human genome. We carry about 100,000 pieces of DNA that came from retroviruses—known as endogenous retroviruses." It then comes as no surprise that "an estimated 5 to 8 percent of the entire human genome" is made up of viral DNA, "several times more DNA that makes up all 20,000 of our protein-coding genes" (Zimmer 2015).

The complicated relation of viruses and their hosts, viruses and their surroundings, viruses and the political economy of travel, food distribution, trade, and commerce is nowhere to be found in the image of the SARS-CoV-2 virus pictured at the beginning of this chapter. The very aspects considered external to the virus (the host, its cells, and its DNA, the outside environment) are erased, leaving the virus suspended in an empty space. However, these same aspects are co-constitutive of the virus. In fact, the isolated container, the virion, only represents one of the several states of the virus (Dupré and Guttiger 2016). The methods and approaches used to study viruses continue to delimit and stabilize an entity otherwise dynamic and in constant dialogue with its milieu.

Classification and taxonomy resort to formal nomenclature based on agreements established by the International Committee on Taxonomy of

Viruses (ICTV). Though this formal taxonomy is constantly changing, its general structure follows groups of related viruses divided into families whose names end in the suffix *viridae* (e.g., Poxviridae). In addition to requiring international coordination, the task of classifying a virus is generally defined as a complex process that can only be achieved today thanks to advanced technologies. Whereas in the past a virus could be only identified by the symptoms it caused, today the "physical structure of a virus particle can be determined directly (by electron microscopy) or indirectly (by biochemical or serological investigation) and is also used in classification" (Cann 2012, 285). Similarly, with the list of malware constantly growing and a potentially global spread, identification and classification by security companies is likewise an international effort. Understandably, information technology is only marginally interested in formal taxonomy that can be easily identified and understood by anyone. In fact, the security industry is more focused on producing solid protection against malware than in communicating its structure and functioning: protecting user operating systems and finding better solutions once the outbreak has occurred is the main goal of security experts. This is demonstrated by the rhetoric used, all focused on protection, securing, shielding, as well as a focus on applications such as antivirus packages and password protection. Generally, understanding classification is only reserved to the insiders, while the user knows malware in general terms (a virus, a work, a spyware, a ransomware), funky names, and popular monikers (I LOVE YOU, Beagle, Doom, etc.).

A study of the status and behavior of viruses leads to an unavoidable acknowledgment of their complexity. However, because of the negotiated processes and the technologies needed to study viruses, shifting the current traditional methods of identification would require a substantial transformation in the way viruses are classified and described. Currently, the disciplines focused on visual display have produced new approaches to better comprehend and to communicate the entangled nature of viruses. In some cases, viruses have been visualized in relation to their environment. However, in most cases, the representation of the virus as "lone wanderer" is still prominent both in the sciences and in the arts.

Onto-Epistemological Dilemmas

The way viruses are visually represented as precisely delineated entities, as well as the iconography behind the lone wanderer, not only perpetuates an interpretation that characterizes them as unities, but also promotes an amplified idea of viruses' agency, as the metaphors used to describe them as war enemies, as parasites, as alien, or as intruders suggest. These metaphors in turn respect the well-established self vs. other tradition to interpret the host (or the body, the self) in opposition to an unknown and usually hostile other.

Similar approaches can be observed in information technology too. As entities that are often compared to biological viruses, computer viruses and other malware are given specific and well-defined sets of characteristics that often remind the viewer of those assigned to biological viruses. Malware is described as a threat to the innocent and vulnerable user: it infects, penetrates, damages, disrupts; its nature is perceived as "other" or as "alien." The tendency to demonize malware by ascribing to it some high level of agency disregards the complex network of connectivity enabling its spread.

The maintenance of these predominant interpretations of viruses has a dual ontological and epistemological origin. First, the materiality of viruses is delimited within well-known parameters, which only partially reflect their actual material structure. Second, it reflects the way that viruses ought to be studied, manipulated, and socio-culturally constructed according to scientific objectives and according to existing socio-cultural and historical abilities to make sense of them. "What is being described by our theories is not nature itself, but our participation within nature" (Barad 2007), Karen Barad observes. The use of war metaphors or the imagination and portrayal of the virus as a self-contained entity are neither products directly deriving from scientific observations, nor mere cultural flourishing resulting from popular perceptions and fears of the virus. The qualities of the entity named virus result from a number of dynamically intersecting factors, or the "intra-action of the observer, the observed, and observing instruments, all of which are 'agential'" (van der Tuin 2012). To put it with Karin Knorr Cetina, we know that the object we call virus is the product of scientific processes, which are socially mediated. In addition, "features of the social world, and more generally of everyday life, become played upon and turned into epistemic devices in the production of science" (Knorr Cetina 1999, 119). In other words, the virus itself, not just the processes leading to its unraveling, is a socio-cultural product. Attempts to define viruses are tied to satisfying a set of goals established by the materiality of the virus itself, as well as by the discipline(s) studying it. The resulting definition and representation of viruses are obtained through a convergence of conventions and established rules, the technologies that apply these rules, and what scientists are interested (or obliged) to reveal through these technologies and rules. These processes are also affected by the potential anxieties that a virus may cause at the popular level, and by the hopes that the results of these processes may also help ease these anxieties.

Providing a well-defined molecular model of a virus or a clear schematics of the way malware functions brings temporary clarity to a fairly elusive agent: the instrument used to examine the agent turns it into an observable, simple, clear object, its boundaries precisely drawn and well defined (Daston and Galison 1992, 116). This presentation, facilitated and performed by mechanical instruments and digital devices, gives a—false and temporary—sense of security, dispelling some of the anxiety that viruses cause, as invisible and unknown entities. To take the virus apart and order it into its discrete molecular parts is not only a practical endeavor but also a mechanism of defense against indeterminacy and the unknown (Frow 2014; Lynch 2006; Robins 1996).

Rendering a virus as a self-contained item has also motivations that are epistemological in nature. Daston and Galison have explained how objectivity may have introduced a set of criteria leading to the acceptance of such rendering as the "correct way to investigate nature" (Daston and Galison 2010, 128). During the scientific revolution "knower and knowledge" became separated. In other words, the object studied becomes something independent from the person who studies it and observes it. What this "separation" means has transformed many times since then, acquiring different values and being attached to different epistemic virtues: for instance, the notion of objective knowledge as a "systematized theoretical account of how the world really is" (51) was first coupled with approaches linked to the moral integrity of the knower, then to the emotionless precision and efficiency of mechanization and quantification.

The increasing faith in quantification has led to today's reliance on mechanically processed, digitally rendered research and on quantification as a way to produce more and precise results (Daston and Galison 1992). Objectivity as we interpret it today connects automatic and mechanical data registration with emotional detachment and with reliability. However, this approach is different from the early mechanized view of the scientific object promoted by the advent of photography. The so-called impartial instrument's gaze is not able to produce a clear view of the virus, in part because of its invisibility, and in part because its complexity needs an interpretive eye. This eye can be seen at work in the way concepts are presented in a precise, clinical, geometrically defined way, to facilitate better discerning and understanding of the object.

Rendering viruses as self-contained, clearly defined, and isolated is a manifestation of this long-lasting tradition. According to Rasmussen, techniques and instruments used in science have to "conform to and yet extend accepted knowledge about living beings" (Rasmussen 1999, 29). To be fully understood and acknowledged, research on viruses (and research in general) cannot use radical innovations or a wholesale revision of research methods, but has to gradually incorporate new findings into a set of "domesticated methods" (Lynch 2006). Thus, although the complex interweaving of viruses with other microorganisms and with the environment surrounding them is largely acknowledged (Dimmock 2001), viruses are still examined as single entities and as fixed objects. Traditional procedures identify them as entities that possess observable characteristics and identifiable inherent capabilities—they are "delimit-able."

The study of viruses includes both observed and constructed elements. The result is a compromise that gathers popular perceptions of viruses and fragments from early literature on plagues and infectious diseases, traditional scientific assumptions and new approaches. While this bargain solution will not fully transmit the complexity of the researched object, it nonetheless abides by the general rules and principles of scientific practice, thus earning ultimate legitimacy (or at least acquiring the right to be a part of a legitimate research practice). An interesting example can be observed in textbooks of introductions to virology: as lengthy discussions provide descriptions of the complex nature of viruses, they must attach this description to schematic language that clearly identifies all the parts involved, as if the virus was a geometrical shape, a building, or a scheme, and accompany it with molecular drawings and schematics that reproduce the same clear-cut and iconic image of the virus molecule I introduced at the beginning of this chapter. For instance, Acheson, in his *Fundamentals of Molecular Virology* (2011), compares the structure of icosahedral viruses to other objects such as a soccer balloon, or architectural forms, such as Buckminster Fuller's iconic geodesic dome.

The ability of viruses to become active when encountering the host, a relational nature, contradicts the practice of isolating them as individual entities. However, scientists researching viruses must employ agreed-on methodologies to guarantee the understanding of their work by other scientists and professionals in their own field and across disciplines. This choice ensures that the presentation of results conforms to the models used in previous studies of microorganisms and provides discrete scientific results and data to legitimize the findings. While the difficult nature of viruses is well-known, not much is being done to find new methods to communicate them. This has little to do with inaccuracy or an inability to incorporate new conceptual understandings of viruses, but has a lot to do with the obligation to respect traditional models while guaranteeing non-ambiguous communication across disciplines. Although hardly reflecting the complex ways in which viruses, humans, and other non-human organisms intersect and coexist, the imperfect, yet popular and somewhat reassuring model of the virus as "lone wanderer" is still the predominant choice: it is relatively easy to identify and it references past research on the subject. Importantly, it makes invisibility visible.

Invisibility

Until the second half of the nineteenth century, the term *virus* was not used as a label for the agent causing a disease. A description of symptoms would be sufficient to name a disease. Even when practitioners were able to determine that infectious diseases were not the product of supernatural forces or miasmatic air particles (Chung-jen Chen 2019), the instruments available could still not detect microbes and viruses. Scientists would therefore attribute their cause to some invisible unidentified agents. In general, Bos observes, there was no immediate interest in isolating and studying the causes of diseases. Curing the disease took priority over studying its specific cause (Bos 1999). Of course, the lack of instruments prevented the identification of any microscopic (or submicroscopic like viruses) infectious agents. Jenner's successful administration of the vaccine against smallpox in 1796 is recognized as a turning point in the acknowledgment of infectious agents (Bos 2000; Lederberg 2000). However, it was only in the 1880s, with Pasteur's experiments on bovine anthrax (Latour 1983), that the first virus was finally transferred to a laboratory and isolated from the myriads of existing microbes.

The identification of the causative agent of tobacco mosaic disease in 1890[2] was a landmark event, and is now acknowledged as the foundation year for virology (Wagner and Hewlett 2004). By distinguishing viruses from bacteria, virology established itself as its own discipline, whose focus was the study of this smaller category of microbes. In the beginning, research conducted focused more on identifying the existence of the causative agent of a disease, rather than analyzing the agent itself. This is clearly illustrated in the focus of the Koch/Lister/Pasteur postulates of germ theory (1. Communicability, 2. Causality, 3. Vitality, and 4. Specificity); on what the germs do, rather than what they are (Ewald 2004).

The first tobacco mosaic virus was only observed in 1935 thanks to the introduction of new methods in crystallography, which allowed scientists to identify the arrangement of atoms beyond the diffraction limit of light, and to the introduction of the electron microscope, which allowed the visualization of objects that were beyond the reach of the classic light microscope. It was then that the morphology of viruses was first observed and distinguished from that of other microorganisms. Before this breakthrough, Lederberg confirms, "most biologists had little, if anything to do with bacteria mid-viruses, or they viewed them as mysterious pre-cellular organisms" (Lederberg 2000). Scientific and technological innovation rapidly increased the amount of information on viruses and allowed their classification according to categories based on functionality and behavior.

Today, viruses are no longer unknown (and unknowable) entities. With techniques such as filtration, micro-crystallography, electron microscopy, live cell imaging, and computer modeling, we have been able to make viruses "partially visible" (Davis 2017; Dimmock 2001; Zimmer 2020).

The ability to visualize viruses at increasingly high resolution and with minimal distortion is considered crucial to understanding them, as is testified by the emphasis on images in research and by the prizes that scientists have shared in the past eighty years. Acheson (2011) explains that virions can be visualized using electron microscopy by negative staining, which "reveals the structure of the virion by the exclusion of electron-absorbing molecules

[2]This event is not to be confused with the later first successful observation of the very virus causing the Tobacco mosaic disease, which happened forty years later in 1935.

such as uranyl acetate" or by positive staining in sections of infected tissue, revealing "proteins, nucleic acids, and lipids." However, these methods can distort or blur structural details of virions. Cryo-electron microscopy, an electron microscopy technique applied to samples cooled to cryogenic temperatures and embedded in an environment of vitreous water (Davis 2017; Krämer 2017), can provide much better resolution and less distortion. The inventors of this method were awarded the Nobel Prize in Chemistry in 2017. The images produced with this technique have extraordinary resolution, thanks to the use of liquid ethane to flash-freeze solutions of proteins, thus "keeping the molecules relatively still when they were hit by electrons" (Cressey and Callaway 2017). This technology has enabled scientists to inspect and measure the molecular structure and composition of viruses.

Despite such advancement, the many assumptions that characterized viruses in previous centuries persist today, not only in the way they are described, but also in the methods used to research them. The nature of viruses is still ambiguous. Can they be classified as organisms? The answer is debated. Most virologists will argue that viruses are passive molecules with two states: inactive (the infectious virus particle) and active (the virus material interacting inside the host cell). Since in their inactive state they only constitute a bundle of genetic material protected by a membrane, they are often qualified as non-living. Although the idea of "life" used to describe viruses has been questioned, it persists.

Do their relational characteristics, that is, their need of a host to reproduce and thrive, make the observation of viruses in isolation somehow obsolete or is it still useful (Cressey and Callaway 2017)? Although a few recent publications have presented a broader view of the nature and the function of viruses and their crucial role in evolutionary processes and in the making of oceans, plants, and the human genome (Mölling 2017; Villarreal 2016), a lot of scholarship and popular science rely on more traditional systems of classification and conceptual descriptions.

Ed Cohen describes viruses as "particular." In fact, they " ... are not universals; they are odd, bizarre, and still familiar; they are individuals and yet they are parts; they are partial—in all possible senses. Moreover, if viruses are particular, it is partly because they are particles. Their particular and particulate nature straddles the cusp of 'life itself,' confusing the very notion of what living means" (Cohen 2011). The fact that they are both particular (they have a "special" status) and particulate (when active, they stretch themselves beyond their own body, merging with something else; yet they do have a separate existence, a body, which they inhabit when inactive) inevitably causes ambiguity. Viruses are described as "infectious agents" by the World Health Organization (WHO), as well as news media and popular science publications. When it is not explained, this description gives the impression that viruses act upon a clueless and victimized population, as if human density and proximity, behavior and the complicated environmental factors causing or favoring the spread of a virus have little import in its outcomes.

Access to and visibility of viruses, or the lack thereof, are considered problems. However, even with the increased information available thanks to enhanced instruments and software, the authoritative words provided by scientific research are often not sufficient to counter the myths created about a microscopic agent that remains invisible to most individuals.

Like biological viruses, computer viruses are invisible. This is not a result of their minuscule size; instead, it is because they have no physical form. They can only be detected by examining computer code. Where researchers have had increasing success over the last thirty years identifying and controlling biological viruses, during this period computer viruses have seemed to have become increasingly more difficult to identify and manage. In fact, they appear to have undergone a process of disappearance.

According to Eric Raymond, computer viruses were not always invisible. This has to do with the increasingly complicated structures that support computers. For Thomas, the degree to which machines are user-friendly is directly proportional to the "degree to which the user is ignorant of the computer's actual operations" (Thomas 2002, 49). The gradual transformation of computers into user-friendly tools had consequences: "the modifications that create a user-friendly environment are usually nothing more than layers which serve to distance the user from the actual operation of the machine" (50). Thus, users are shielded from having to worry about difficult programming. Software and visually immediate or graphic user interface applications (GUI) are doing the work for them.

While the shift "from computation-intensive design to presentation-intensive design" (Raymond 1999) promoted computers' accessibility and usability by allowing computer illiterates to operate increasingly powerful machines, it also made them more complex. Thomas explains how "dragging and dropping a file from one folder to the other still executes a copy command, but the user never sees that part of the process" (Thomas 2002, 52). As extra functions and features were added to the operating system that initially constituted the computer core, the user's awareness of the existence and the role of these functions and features faded.

As a result of the complexity of personal computers and the proliferation of graphic-intensive programs on top of the existing platform, it is no longer necessary—or at least it is no longer perceived as necessary—for users to have programming skills or knowledge related to the operating system. Computer viruses, programmed by means of the same basic code that composes the computer core, stay outside of the familiar interfaces familiar to computer users. As a result, computer viruses disappear from the sight of the average user, who increasingly thinks of them as invisible, uncatchable, and, thus, mysterious.

Like viruses that cause biological infections, computer viruses cannot be immediately detected. Discovery of the presence of a computer virus occurs when the user is alerted by their computer's antivirus software, or if the computer starts malfunctioning for no apparent reason. The actual virus cannot be observed by users unless the user is trained in computer coding. What becomes obvious is not the very substance of a computer virus, but the effects produced by code when the virus is executed.

The difficulty in visualizing and defining viruses has several significant implications. Viruses are caught into an onto-epistemological dilemma: how do we best characterize them? Despite their—abstract, unstable, and shifting—nature, it is imperative to define them. The inability to do so accurately is both due to their ontological peculiarities and the epistemological framework that insist on examining them using traditional perspectives for clarity, practicality, and reassurance. While admittedly some approaches are old-fashioned, other methods predominant today are difficult to leave behind because they have been part of a long tradition of scientific research. Importantly, popular beliefs cannot be ignored.

Entangled Realities—A Different View on Viruses

Although largely to be considered creative renditions, there exist a handful of notable examples that acknowledge the fact that molecular life and information technologies, viruses, bacteria, and multicellular organisms alike are made up of internal processes and interactions between symbiotic and non-symbiotic constituents, leading to intricate ecologies and powerful connectedness. Microbiologist and scientific illustrator David Goodsell has been drawing and painting brightly colored scientific illustrations of microscopic life and mechanisms able to convey the relational processes of transmission of viruses and bacteria and the molecular richness of the cell. A radically different example is Greg Bear's literary account of a digital machinery turning into an organism in the short story *Blood Music*, which he then turned into a full novel, and, later into a series of novels involving viruses (both informational and biological) imagined as evolutionary machines.

In the book *The Machinery of Life*, David Goodsell describes the world as "overflowing with the diversity of life" (Goodsell 2010, 7). This diversity is woven together by countless loops, threads, and connections: "By examining the plants, birds, and animals that surround us, scientists have discovered that you and I are directly related to every other living thing on the Earth" (Goodsell 2010, 1). For Goodsell, all items in this world share one single history: at the molecular level, everything is made of not very dissimilar matter: in fact, "when you look in the microscope, you will find that all living organisms are composed of cells, and that the cells in a tree look amazingly similar to the cells in your own hand" (Goodsell 2010, 2).

Combined in different ways, he argues, matter forms entwined molecular machines. Goodsell's illustrations of microscopic organisms and biological phenomena (molecular machines) have both scientific and educational goals: in addition to showing a precise rendering of the complexity constituting a molecular machine, he immerses them in the rich context hosting them, in order to reveal their relations and interdependence.

His book displays a heterogeneous collection of illustrations, including a range of molecular phenomena, water molecules, proteins, ribosomes, bacteria, and viruses. The illustrations are meticulously drawn, created upon careful comparison of different protein models from the Protein Data Bank (PDB), and other crystallography samples (Wellcome Collection n.d.).

Founded in 1971, the PDB database is a worldwide open-source archive for macromolecular structure data, collecting digitized molecular structures obtained from chemical analysis, microscopy and X-ray data, and other sources. Scientists format their lab results and make them available to other scientists and to the public. In addition to uploading data for the purpose of research sharing, the PDB also has educational purposes, providing programs and tutorials to the public at large and to young visitors. Goodsell has been contributing to this database both as a scientist and as an illustrator.

Besides their aesthetic singularity manifested in the use of a distinctive brightly colored palette, his illustrations are quite innovative: whereas models and visualizations typically display molecular components as separate items—in the case of proteins, as disembodied ribbons—Goodsell reconnects the parts as if he was reassembling a puzzle, collecting and recombining them to reconstruct a whole image, which contains information obtained from several sources. The result captures "the current state of knowledge" and shows the subject (a virus, a cell, a bacteria) as well as its context (Goodsell 2020). For instance, we see illustrations of the agents of immune system piercing a bacterial cell wall, the cycle of a poliovirus while entering a cell and releasing its active components inside the cell, an influenza virus budding from the surface of cells not as single proteins, or as isolated virus parts, but as dynamic agents making their way across very dense and populated environments.

In all illustrations, viruses and proteins' parts appear sharply identified—their contours well-traced—to add clarity and depth to the soupy environment that contains them. Knowing the difficulty of making sense of molecular life when it is not possible to detect it using the naked eye, all components are reproduced with a consistent scale in mind, in order to allow the observer to not only acquire a sense of the real size of the molecules, but to also compare different molecular landscapes. Establishing a consistent scale enables the reader to compare, for example, *E. coli* bacteria, a large organism, to the polio virus and the rhinovirus, two small viruses, or to identify lipids and proteins inside the cell. Goodsell uses different color schemes to help readers better read the images. Although the colors chosen to depict, for example, ribosomes, viral RNA, and lipid molecules are admittedly arbitrary, they are consistently utilized throughout the body of illustrations contained in the book. Also, they add a bit of dramatic contrast to help the narrative.

Goodsell's goal is to "show the whole story," that is, how everything is deeply connected and undergoes different processes and stages of development (SciArt Initiative 2020). Scientists and individuals with a basic knowledge of biology know, of course, the interactions occurring in the microbial world, and that models and renderings, though simplified, are useful in examining specific molecular landscapes. For Goodsell, it is important to circulate illustrations of entire phenomena, to remind the public of the articulations involved in the life cycle of the cell and of the molecular world. The clarity of his illustrations is not only beautifully crafted, but also very accessible.

In early 2020, he released two paintings portraying respectively the coronavirus "just entering the lungs, surrounded by mucus secreted by respiratory cells" (Figure 2) and the coronavirus life cycle, showing "a cross section through a cell infected with a coronavirus such as SARS-CoV-2" (Figure 3). Both paintings are now displayed on the main page, as well as on the educational section of the RCSB (Research Collaboratory for Structural Bioinformatics, the organization responsible for the management of PDB) Protein Data Bank (PDB).

The educational version of the painting reveals in great detail its process of creation, from the original microscopy and the archival material it was modeled from, to how each part contained in the virus and around the virus was drawn and colored. To distinguish the cell particles from the virus, Goodsell used different shades of blue (cell) and purple/pink (viral molecules): the contrasting colors show how viruses and cells intersect and interact with each other. Goodsell tried different combinations of colors before reaching a satisfactory image. He describes how every time colors and contrast are changed, a different set of elements would emerge: for example, using a different set of colors would underscore the way in which the external vesicles of the virus protect and allow its content to circulate. Goodsell explains how posting the paintings in the educational section of PDB was important as an outreach strategy and to understand how the public reacted to and comprehended the illustrations. A 101 Outreach coloring model released in May 2020 that encouraged the public at large to create their favorite coronavirus color scheme and to post it on twitter proved a successful discussion piece (SciArt Initiative 2020).

Goodsell's paintings both demonstrate and question the onto-epistemological foundations underlying the conceptual interpretation of viruses. While his illustrations strive to present the whole story, to highlight the connectedness of the parts and the busyness of the environment surrounding cells and viruses, he still carefully separates and colorizes the parts for clarity, calling them molecular machines. The latter is a term recently embraced by the biological sciences: typically adopted in education

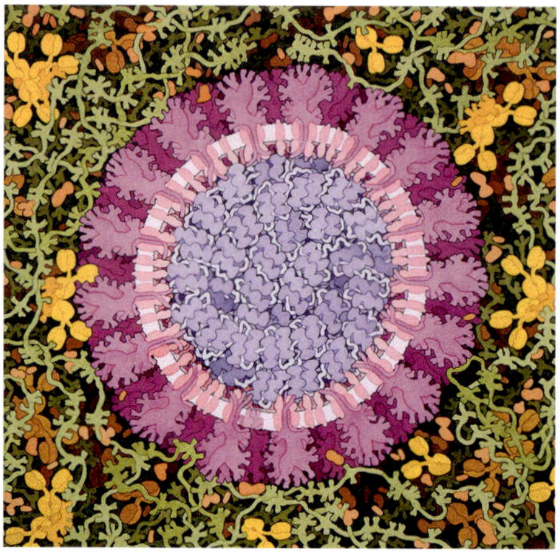

FIGURE 2 *Illustration by David S. Goodsell, RCSB Protein Data Bank; doi: 10.2210/rcsb_pdb/goodsell-gallery-019. This painting depicts a coronavirus just entering the lungs, surrounded by mucus secreted by respiratory cells, secreted antibodies, and several small immune systems proteins. The virus is enclosed by a membrane that includes the S (spike) protein, which will mediate attachment and entry into cells, M (membrane) protein, which is involved in organization of the nucleoprotein inside, and E (envelope) protein, which is a membrane channel involved in budding of the virus and may be incorporated into the virion during that process. The nucleoprotein inside includes many copies of the N (nucleocapsid) protein bound to the genomic RNA.*

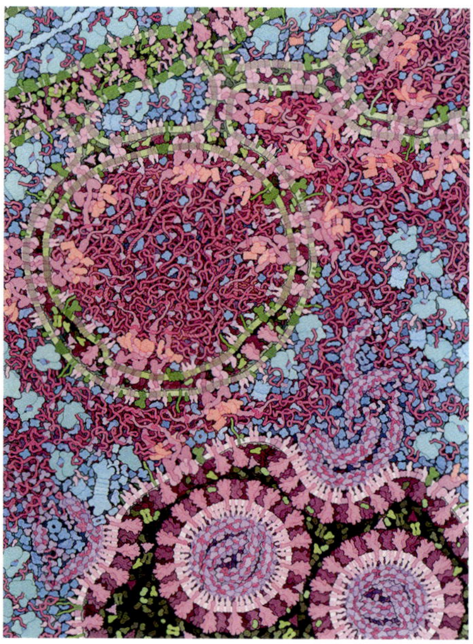

FIGURE 3 *David S. Goodsell, RCSB Protein Data Bank; doi: 10.2210/rcsb_pdb/goodsell-gallery-023.*

to facilitate better comprehension of the parts comprising cells and microorganisms, it is also the result of an engineering turn in biology, that is, a general trend to adopt engineering methods and approaches to study biology (Myers 2015; Roosth 2017). Goodsell's illustrations use the style and the metaphorical language promoted by this trend, while introducing a new iconography that reveals connectedness and entanglement rather than separation, geometry, and machine-like rendering. The illustration of SARS CoV-2 still highlights the virus as separated from its environment. Yet the boundaries of the virus have become looser and now it comes in two versions, one for each state.

Currently, there are many science fiction novels and short stories involving viruses as their protagonists. However, most of them present computer viruses as exclusively informational. Greg Bear's 1983 short story *Blood Music*, later to become an award-winning novel, is one of the exceptions. The kind of virus he described is technically not informational, but is mediated through information. This makes it particularly interesting. In the short story, a radical experiment leads the protagonist Virgil Ulam to inject himself with biological computers based on his own lymphocytes (which he calls noocytes). Once inside his body, the noocytes multiply and evolve, altering their own genetic material and becoming self-aware. This results in a pandemic in which information/biological hybrid engines merge with humans and non-human alike, transforming the way they communicate.

Bear's visionary scenario breaks with at least two well-established discourses: first, with the idea that cross-contamination between humans, non-humans, and machines is impossible. Second, that it will be catastrophic. In *Blood Music*, this process is neither apocalyptic nor pessimistic. It is true that computer viruses will probably never infect any human beings. However, biology and information technology have been in a constant dialogue for decades. Such relation has been rarely studied, as there is currently a gap between disciplines close to media studies or network cultures—which have focused exclusively on informational networks—and other disciplines such as science studies and science and technology studies. Bear's story makes us think of useful comparisons between information and biology by showing just how their functioning relies on multiple processes and intersections.

In the novel, the virus-like engines that the protagonist decides to inject into his own body smoothly (not violently) merge with their hosts—they don't attack them—providing apparent improvements (not destruction), and promoting previously unimaginable interpersonal and interspecies communications (not interruption). In describing the relationship between the noocytes and their diverse hosts, Bear emphasizes the reality of their coexistence. Bear's scenario is exceptional in that it eschews human exceptionalism and rejects the usual portrayal of viruses as evil threats to the humans, who are classically seen as the protagonists and the unlucky victims. The way that information and biology come to merge in the story is not painless: the protagonist experiences some deep anxiety when he is faced with the initial effects of the virus. However, this anxiety is soon replaced by a dialogue, as an acknowledgment of the inevitable symbiotic relationship emerging from the intersection and the fusion of the virus and the human body. These are Virgil-now-turned-virus's final words: "All my hatred and fear is gone now I leave them—us—with only one question. How many times has this happened, elsewhere? Travelers never came through space to visit the Earth. They had no need. They had found universes in grains of sand" (Bear 1983).

Goodsell's illustrations teeming with particles and Bear's terse description of machine-to-human infiltration/repopulation are exceptions, not the norm. Their perspectives show different ways to contemplate viruses. Indeed, viruses neither exist in isolation nor are they exclusively acting as the enemy.

Taxonomy and Classification of Viruses

As partially living entities, viruses do not fit conventional taxonomy systems inspired by Linnaeus and based on the Darwinian principle of common descent for organisms and plants. These types of classifications assume that, although evolving over a time span, species are comprised of stable and self-sufficient organisms (van Regenmortel and Fauquet 2000). As entities whose existence mutates once in contact with a host and that can be studied mostly in relation to it, viruses may become difficult to classify, unless one ranks them in a specific moment of their development. Siddell, among other virologists, argues that "the spectrum of genetic diversity for viruses is a continuum, so that any attempt to divide them into different categories will not be sustainable" (Siddell 2018). It comes as no surprise then that some scholars have declared taxonomy "an empty exercise." Interest in taxonomy in the general areas of microbiology and virology has apparently been in decline, becoming an activity basically carried out by volunteers (Simmonds et al. 2017). However, Siddell continues, taxonomy should not be abandoned: the discipline is constantly developing to adapt to new findings and it might ultimately help better understand the origins, scope, and impact of virus evolution. More specifically, the scope and range of taxonomy have transformed in recent years, shifting from classifying viruses that cause damage to humans, plants, and animals to virus discovery for environmental and evolutionary research.

The front page of the ICTV (International Committee on Taxonomy of Viruses) database warns:

> Taxonomy lies at the uneasy interface between biology and logic. The processing of information follows somewhat different rules in these two systems and the role of taxonomy is to reconcile them as tidily as possible. To this end, the International Union of Microbiological Societies

> (IUMS) charged the International Committee on Taxonomy of Viruses (ICTV) with the task of developing, refining, and maintaining a universal virus taxonomy (ICTVdb, n.d.). The type of classification mostly agreed upon is a hybrid one: a combination of two main methods, the Baltimore Classification System and the ICTV classification guidelines.
>
> (Buchen-Osmond 2003; M. H. V. van Regenmortel and Mahy 2004)

The Baltimore Classification System identifies seven groups of viruses marked by Roman numerals, based on their morphological composition and nucleic acid type. The ICTV classification system is superimposed on the former and derives from the existing classic taxonomy: its function is to allocate virus species within major morphological groups and by their phenotypes. Viruses are usually distinguished by status, between those that reside inside a cell (intracellular) and those floating outside of a cell (extracellular). If a virus is extracellular, it is called a *virion*, that is, a virus in a non-active state or not attached to a host. A *virion* contains a protein coating called a capsid, which surrounds the core of the virus containing the nucleic acid (either DNA or RNA). Once identified into different species, *virions* are subdivided by mode of replication, host organisms, and the type of viruses they cause.

The fact that there is a need to combine two different systems is important. It is a necessity to not only define viruses as isolated objects (as the Baltimore System does), but also to classify them (as the ICTV system does) as entities that are both linked to their hosts and to the diseases they cause, a condition necessary to qualify them as active.

The relational nature of biological viruses forces the taxonomic system to equally account for both the cause (the virus as object) and effect (the disease this virus causes), and to consider the linkage between any virus strain and its host during the naming process. For example, within Class I of viruses the family poxviridae carries the term "pox," indicative of the physical or macro-manifestation of a particular virus upon the host (through the appearance of poxes on the host's skin). The same term is then used to name the disease that is caused (smallpox, chickenpox); the influenza virus is classified as a Class IV, or ssRNA negative-strand viruses, and is named Orthomyxoviridae, after myxa, meaning "mucus." Recently, the family of Coronaviridae (Class IV under the Baltimore system) has received a lot of attention. The Coronaviridae Study Group determined that SARS-CoV-2 belongs to an existing species, the severe acute respiratory syndrome-related coronavirus containing three different viruses responsible for the 2020 COVID-19 pandemic, the 2003 outbreak of SARS, and the 2012 of MERS.

The particular method adopted by the ICTV associates the disease caused by the virus with the active agent. A recent development in the classification of viruses follows the increasing amount of metagenomic data that has become available about viruses. A panel of scientists argued that "the number and diversity of viral sequences that are identified in metagenomic data far exceeds that of experimentally characterized virus isolates" (Simmonds et al. 2017). This prompted them to propose that viruses that are known only from metagenomic data be incorporated into the official classification scheme of the ICTV. This turn toward acknowledging the complex diversity that characterizes what we know of viruses today falls in line with new directions in the taxonomy of species biology: Dayrat, for example, proposes an integrative approach to taxonomy that takes into account the current complexity of species biology by studying the units of life's diversity from multiple and complementary perspectives (phylogeography, comparative morphology, population genetics, ecology, development, behavior, etc.) (Dayrat 2005).

The acknowledgment of the diversity of viruses and their relational features has not changed the way in which they are classified by applying the same taxonomic system used for other organisms. The choice is dictated by consistency and functionality but, as we have seen early in this chapter, it also ends up affecting the way we perceive viruses.

Similar generalizations and difficulties of classifications can be observed in the treatment of computer viruses. Computing experts become aware of new malware when it has already spread. At this point, the focus is not on classification but on security, as the main goal of the antivirus industry is defeating viruses rather than thoroughly studying them. This focus is due in part to the speed at which viruses, worms, spyware, and many other types of malware are released: the antivirus industry is on constant call as security threats are always around the corner. In this context, the classification of malware is seen as something of minor value: although classification is needed for research purposes, it is mostly developed as something temporary, used to facilitate the early detection and labeling of a virus by the security software, which in turn allows the user of infected software to apply the right antivirus product.

Currently, there are only a few organizations that focus on computer virology reports. Organizations such as EICAR (established in 1991 as the European Institute for Computer Antivirus Research) produce periodical updates on the most current computer malware in a given period. Since new computer viruses are discovered at a very fast rate, each antivirus company proceeds independently, by what Sarah Gordon, in an early article, called "interim naming" (Gordon 2002), that is, by applying a temporary name to each newly detected virus. To explain this tendency, a spokesperson from WildList, an organization that collects data on the detection of viruses from individuals and antivirus companies and monitors new computer viruses (interestingly, they describe the active malware as being "in the wild"), once offered the following example to explain the lack of interest in classification for the sake of research:

> There's a weed growing in my back yard. I call it Lamb's Quarters. It's a very common weed, and is also known as Goose Foot, Pig Weed, Sow Bane, and a few other things. I don't know what it's called in South

> Africa, Hungary, India, or Taiwan, but I'm sure it has lots and lots of names. I'm not a biological researcher. I'm just an end user. I yank the weeds and mow the lawn. I call it Lambs Quarters and don't care what it's called in Hungary.
>
> (from a now removed page of the Wildlist.org 2006[3])

In this context, the naming of viruses is considered irrelevant for users, as their preoccupation lies primarily on keeping their computer clean and removing any unwanted malware (Gordon 2002). In addition to being relatively new, the discipline that examines computer viruses is fast transforming and lies in a constant state of emergency. The primary goal is the speedy resolution of security problems. Since antivirus products are usually customer-oriented, the need for accuracy in naming and classification for research purposes is not deemed vital. Gordon argued that while science has relied on a "..rich amount of reference samples and on an already existing sample based naming scheme, the problem with applying this approach in the antivirus world has been the lack of a reference collection or even a central naming body" (2002, 4).

In 1999, Vassily Bontchev had already made a controversial presentation at the computer virus bulletin conference, questioning the relevance of organizations such as the WildList, which rely on volunteers to detect malware and publish new findings only once a month, too late to be of any use. Marx and Dessmann (2007) point out that in addition to its slowness, the WildList only contains "intentionally malicious software which is able to self-replicate by infecting other files (viruses) and PCs in a network environment (worms)." However, malware is not always malicious: it can be faulty code causing disastrous consequences. In addition, the types of malware roaming our networks today are highly diversified, comprising bots, spyware and adware, backdoors, memory worms, etc.

The lack of interest in classification and taxonomy goes hand in hand with the absence of computer literacy amongst users causing code to disappear, and by blackboxing, which often limits user access to encoded and encrypted content. Commercial antivirus software provides no specific information about the cause of a computer malfunction, nor does it give the user any instruction on virus removal. Users are not encouraged to modify the standardized configuration of their antivirus package and are simply prompted to authorize periodical and automated security updates designed to prevent generic malware intrusions.

The disempowering of the user contributes to the strengthening of the assumption that computer viruses are mysterious entities created by some malicious agencies. Users are not only dissuaded from self-educating, they are also discouraged from taking responsibility for their online behavior

---

[3]The WildList used to be active between 1993 and 2016. Today most of its pages and references have been removed. However, the list of viruses "in the wild" is updated regularly by a long list of contributors around the world.

and for their very contribution in spreading malware. Once user agency is dismissed, the battle against malware is given over to the antivirus corporations, which are able to further the narrative that all problems relating to computer malfunctioning must be invariably ascribed to the evil action of some computer virus, and that only they can correct the problem.

Viruses are often better known not by their technical name, but by their "media name" or their "aliases." Raiu (2002) notes: "When the 'VBS/VBSWG.J' virus appeared, the media decided to call it by a more appealing name, *Anna Kournikova*, after the JPEG file that the email carrying the virus claimed to contain." However, and despite the easy identification, popular or media names are often rejected and dismissed by antivirus programmers. In fact, antivirus software vendors often establish their own classification and naming systems, in part because of practical reasons, in part to discredit virus writers: "Dubbing the malicious code 'Melissa,' after a Miami stripper, flies in the face of many naming conventions that antivirus companies follow today. For example, using the name provided by the virus writer is avoided at all costs to avoid bestowing credibility upon the author" (Marx and Dessmann 2007). Security analysts and researchers proposed a variety of methods to classify viruses using morphology, increased complexity (from simple to polymorphic), target discovery, etc. (Spafford 1994; Szor 2005). However, these methods of classification seem to fall short because of their focus on discriminating between viruses and non-viruses.

To solve this problem, Webster and Malcolm proposed a new method based on "whether any of the reproductive actions [of computer viruses] are afforded by other entities, or not" (M. Webster and Malcolm 2018). This method draws on Gibson's theory of affordances, which defines affordance as an ecological theory of perception: "animals perceive objects in their environment, to which their instincts or experience attach a certain significance based on what that object can afford (i.e., do for) the animal." The model is relational by nature, assuming that malware can activate and is most effective when it encounters a system that can accommodate it. Typically, the model compares computing to a biological environment, illustrating how this comparison is not just metaphorical but material as well. Importantly, it shows how alternatives to traditional classification models that reflect more complex network scenarios and biological entanglement are indeed possible.

How to Describe Complexity?

Becoming aware of the challenges in using ready-made categories to classify viruses may teach us something about current onto-epistemological tenets in culture and technoscience in general. Michel Foucault offered ways to map the intricate connection of forces that may lead to different understandings and conceptualizations of the world. This framework may help understand how multiple ways of qualifying and describing viruses are the result of them being simultaneously repositories, perpetuators, and generators of discursive formations.

Foucault famously argued that discourse proceeds by ruptures, whose micro-narratives reoccur in different places and at different times, taking on different meanings according to the contexts in which they locate themselves. Discourse takes different trajectories, which connect and intersect in non-linear ways, forming series that lie at different conceptual and disciplinary planes. These series are "juxtaposed with one another, follow one another, overlap and intersect, without one being able to reduce them to a linear schema" (Foucault 1989a, 9). Viruses (when classified as delimited and self-contained objects) are not the sole enablers of the discourse that characterizes them, as discourse is never the product of a single entity (i.e., viruses, with their inherent qualities), but involves this very entity in its relation to what is around it. This discourse comes from the interaction of viruses as objects with society, technologies, networks, etc. As the product of a diverse and multifaceted variety of interactions and interpretations, this discourse cannot be interpreted as unified, but something that takes on different forms depending on the quality and variety of interactions. Foucault suggested that one of the possible ways to map such moments should not be limited to understanding how discourses record or memorize documents, but also how they "transform them into monuments" (9), implying that the process of building discourse, rather than the result of this process, is what is crucial.

Foucault and other scholars who have dedicated themselves to understanding how humans (as a general category, or *anthropós*) have conceptualized and used the world to their benefit have critiqued conventional approaches that see the result of the interactions between phenomena and their cultural and social impact as a constellation of usually self-contained and distinct (yet dynamic) objects and phenomena. However, the formation of the technologies by which nature and culture interact in the expression and socio-cultural construction of viruses cannot be conceptualized as a static constellation, as Foucault seems to describe, but must be understood more dynamically, as a series of temporary coagulations of processes.

Karen Barad argues that nature, or whatever we consider to be nature, always ends up embedded in a complex ecological system comprised of nature itself, the instruments that analyze it, individuals, ideas regarding nature, etc. Her theoretical analysis of agential realism here elucidates how "the dynamism of naturalcultural practices and matter" (Barad 2007, 135) is implicit in viruses. In fact, nature contains matter and meaning simultaneously (56). The two (or the many) cannot be separated and/or analyzed separately as they are in constant co-evolution and in co-relation with the surrounding environment, be it comprised of humans and non-humans, bacteria, diatoms, plants, or bits and circuits.

Following Barad's explanation then, "words and things" are not located in a relation of correspondence. In fact, to research "a causal explanation of how discursive practices are related to material phenomena" one should be "shifting the focus from the nature of representations to the nature of scientific practice" (45). It is important to clarify that here representation does not refer to visual representation (or not exclusively to it), but to a habit of understanding things as static, as definite objects. Barad's performative approach attempts to capture the complexity of phenomena through a dynamic view. Her goal is to cease obsessing over one specific subject and look around for the ways in which this object is constantly transformed by establishing relations with and encountering what surrounds it. This approach is what she calls realism, a "commitment to accounting for the material nature of practices and how (and as) they come to matter," that is, an attention to the way that discourses, materiality, and subjective interpretation are dynamically and continuously modulated.

The vitality that characterizes discursive practices and the material world, and in this case facilitates the mobility of viruses and the transfering of their connotations from one domain to the other, does not happen as a plain connection, a static point of intersection on a grid, but a moving connection that constantly fluctuates and recombines. We can consider the qualities manifested by, and ascribed to, viruses as not fixed but constantly negotiated through their own material position and present state, through the disparate discourses that attempt to tame their indeterminacy or to fit them into categories and constraints, and through the instrumentalization of these qualities and their potentials.

According to Barad, addressing the significance of matter and the role of the "material," as Foucault did in forming or affecting specific phenomena or events, is useful because it acknowledges the existence of an effective relation between human and non-human: viruses are understood and theorized in this way because of the convergence of certain traditions, technologies, and beliefs. However, the materiality of objects—in the case of viruses, technology, code, and biological particles—and their dynamic relations with the human (a room crowded with people, or users exchanging messages) and non-human actors (software and files in a computer, the environmental conditions of a neighborhood or a city) are equally important factors to consider in determining the configuration and the trajectory of viral agents. Foucault's analysis never abandons the assumption that human actors ultimately decide the direction and the outcome of phenomena. Barad acknowledges the role of the human in its own differential constitution and its positioning among other entities, but "takes issue" with human exceptionalism, especially with the idea that while discourses incorporate human and non-human intersections, the human is the main actor responsible for piecing together and making sense of such intersections.

Keeping this dynamic and non-anthropocentric approach in mind, what would a new method of analysis, representation, or interpretation of the complex configuration and behavior of viruses be? Could the complex convergence of multiple forces, changing qualities, and human and non-human encounters be incorporated into one artifact, into one single document, or using one medium? Let's take, for instance, the way that a virus is represented as an individual and isolated object seemingly detached from its surroundings. We can approach this artifact as a product of a series of chemical and digitization processes, analog and digital technologies, opinions, studies, individuals before reaching its final appearance. Instead of accepting one interpretation, we could become aware of the layers that have converged into producing this artifact; we could reflect on the political and disciplinary compromises, the material difficulties, the obligations made by pre-existing rules, the scientific canons and methods that scientists had to respect (Stengers 2010). But what if we learnt to consider the virus not as a finite object, but as a dynamic entity immersed in, and coexisting with, all the richness surrounding it? Would we be able, as Barad proposes, to seize its onto-epistemological complexity? As I reflect on this possibility, I am drawn back to Goodsell's painting and Bear's writing as they propose to embrace, even if partially, even if temporarily, the ambiguous ontology and epistemological multiplicity of viruses. Looking at these examples may actually inspire the unlocking of new methods that still acknowledge the long tradition of classification and taxonomy, while communicating more nuanced portraits of viral agents.

2

Navigating the Unfamiliar: Strategies of Coping

Modeling Viral Realities

"Models have become reality in the making," Thierry Bardini (2016) argues. A model, whether analog or digital, "is the means we use to ignore what we cannot understand and to consider what we can understand. The use of models allows us to simulate unfamiliar problems by replacing the unfamiliar with the familiar" (Bardini 2016, 380). Whether visually representing, classifying, or describing viruses, there seems to be a preoccupation in making them a bit more familiar to scientists and to a non-scientific public.

As models and renditions make viruses more legible, the colors and shades, the geometric forms they display and other qualities employed in these renditions appear to undermine the reality they represent. In the previous chapter, we have seen the tendency to represent viruses as isolated entities, or as lone wanderers, and the fact that informational and biological viruses are often encased in suspiciously well-defined visual structures. The recurrence of predetermined, assumed, and discrete characterizations expresses a desire to produce clarity without violating the rules and obligations that govern scientific and technical knowledge.

These representations inevitably retain some preconceived ideas derived from popular culture and historical narratives; they incorporate fears and anxieties deriving from present or recent incidents; and they include conventional knowledge, established scientific protocols, and stylistic conventions. Specifically, the way in which viruses are set in a particular taxonomical order reveals a desire to reduce them to entities that can be measurable, contained, and somehow controlled. At the same time, it reflects the important legacy of the early conflation of information and biology. In this chapter, I will focus on this important relationship, which scholars like Donna Haraway, Eve Keller, Judith Roof, and Lily Kay, to name a few, have often described as a marriage, an implosion, and as a busy relationship.

When we see an image of a virus we rarely speculate about what process has led to this product. This process is the product of an interesting circular exchange involving information and biology. We should consider that ideas regarding the circulation and exchange of concepts across the realms of information and biology have origins in the drive to control molecular material as information. Shannon and Weaver's mathematical theory of communication and the genomic turn that has dominated the second half of the twentieth century have taught us to think of the biological and the informational as realms whose principles can be compared and to a certain extent made interchangeable. In fact, be they genes, or bits of code, both digital machines and biological beings are made to be measured by discrete packets. I say "made to be measured" because it is thanks to the application of arbitrary and agreed-upon parameters, and thanks to the practice of modeling, as Bardini suggested early on, that the two domains could be compared. The introduction and pervasiveness of technologies that collect information as discrete data and digitize the biological to make it machine readable and translatable have certainly intensified the exchanges further. Given the benefits that this connection would generate in terms of material and genetic control, that is, in terms of the ability to predict, model, modulate, and manage complex phenomena, the comparison has become, as Lily Kay has suggested, "commonsensical" (Kay 2000, 19; 1997).

Today, there exists a complicated debate that only implicitly involves the relationship between information and biology. Relatively recent disciplines such as bioinformatics, for instance, confirm the extent to which biology is being translated into quantified computational material as the result of a need to sort through the sheer amount of data produced through research, and as a way of knowing that has become increasingly dominant (Thacker 2004). The recent trend in studying and teaching biology through the lens of engineering can be considered the culmination of this tendency, and it is demonstrated by the way in which biology is said to have transformed thanks to "molecular and genomics revolutions ... by making biological 'parts' and 'components' available to manipulation at the molecular scale"(Myers 2015). The rise of synthetic biology has generated the concept of bio-bricks, that is, the practice of thinking of biological material as a combination of interchangeable—Lego like—building blocks, as well as the reformulation of the life sciences as disciplines directly connected to, and shaped by, engineering.

These developments have further blurred the boundaries between the two domains (Myers 2014; Roosth 2017). The engineering turn has brought us attempts to recreate, optimize, modify, and edit biological material, or to "make life better, one part at a time" as Drew Endy, a pioneer of synthetic biology has argued. According to this approach, viruses and bacteria could be modified and reprogrammed, and organisms can be modified to express different characteristics. Yet, while this turn makes it seem very easy at the theoretical level to "crack the code" of bacteria, viruses, and other more complex biological materials, including human cells, it has proven to be much more complicated once the theory is transferred to the experimental "wet" level.

While it seems that until recently most enthusiasm has been concentrated on turning biology into information, the exponential development of information systems into AI applications has revealed a new, never-before-acknowledged complexity. The assumption that it is possible to control and measure the intricate matter of life by means of information technologies and digitization techniques has been reciprocated by a tendency to ascribe biological features to information and by the realization that what we call information is increasingly achieving higher levels of material and existential sophistication. The latter is substantiated by the proliferation of big data and by the growth of whole disciplines dedicated to facilitating the reading and artfully displaying of information, such as data science and data visualization (boyd and Crawford 2012).

Computer and biological viruses, as well as other viral phenomena, especially when they are examined side by side, exemplify the ways information and biology may engage in mutual exchanges: qualities are shared across the two domains, methods of analysis are shared across disciplines, language becomes interchangeable. The viral becomes an overarching category that not only enables viruses to exceed pre-assigned boundaries and preconceived categories, but also embodies an epistemological and disciplinary convergence.

In *The Century of the Gene*, Eve Keller shows how the idea of the gene, an abstract concept and much contested biomolecular component, has not only been heavily affected by discourse (Keller 2000); it has also come to acquire multiple meanings (Myers 2015). Judith Roof adds that "when the basic term for an immense set of practices and concepts [such as the concept of the gene] begins to function as just a single term for many different processes—language becomes an impediment instead of a means of communication" (Roof 2007, 11). The language used to describe biological and informational viruses and other viral phenomena that are technically not viruses but behave like them presents similar dynamics. Descriptive terms adopted to define very different viruses may have been historically useful to identify and take precautions against their spread and the formation of epidemics. At that time, these terms were used to provide clarity and impact. For instance, the use of metaphors and verbs that attributed (evil) agency to an entity that until recently was—neither molecularly, nor visually—identifiable had an impact on the way populations have responded and reacted to epidemics. Once more information was known about viruses and different ailments were attributed to distinct microscopic agents, the metaphors, figurations, stories, and myths that had been created in the past and had made their way into popular culture and fiction did not disappear, even when scientific evidence refuted early beliefs. These same narratives and metaphors were then employed to identify malware.

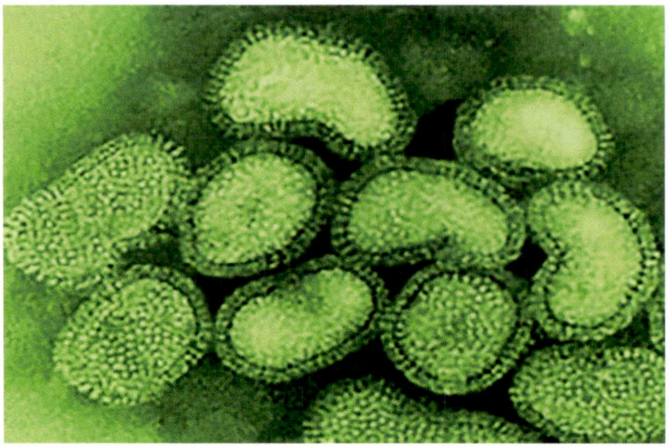

FIGURE 4 *Electron microscopy image of an influenza virus. Photograph by Dr. L Stannard. © University of Cape Town (2023).*

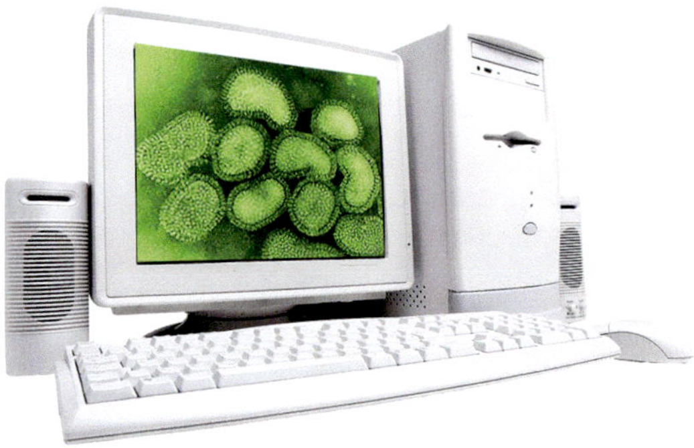

FIGURE 5 *Popular image representing a virus infecting a computer. The image of influenza virus is used to picture a computer virus. Image courtesy of the author.*

Given the trend toward producing digital, geometric images of biological viruses, it should not come as a surprise to see colorized images of a virus (Figure 4) magically appear on a computer screen (Figure 5) to signal the presence of a computer virus or to indicate an infected computer. The computer has literally caught the flu. In this case, the hypothetical morphology and behavior of a computer virus are directly borrowed from the visual vocabulary of microbiology and virology. Why not make such analogy, when both the methodological process (with its increasing rationalization), and the technologies used (with their direction toward geometry), encourage it?

Virology and epidemiology have shown that viruses do not really attack a host, and the immune system is not a citadel to be defended, as some early immunological theories would affirm; computer viruses, since their theorization and definition, have always depended on network density and interactions in order to function. However, in both cases, older vocabulary is being liberally used. As I will explain in later chapters, this vocabulary is not solely used to communicate information, but is the result of, and caters to, emotional responses.

Uncanny Similarities

Consider two radically different images, respectively the work of interdisciplinary artist and sculptor Luke Jerram (Figure 6) and designer and programmer Alex Dragulescu (Figure 7). The first one is a glass sculpture of the molecular model of the Avian Flu (also known as H5N1). The second one is a digital illustration of MyDoom, a computer worm affecting Windows operating systems. The two works demonstrate the extent to which methods and conventional forms of representation not only are preserved in radically different renditions of viruses, but they are also exchanged across the realms of biology (Jerram) and information (Dragulescu). In both cases, "making familiar" acquires a crucial significance for opposite reasons. Generalizations are used out of necessity and as a strategy to either construct a material, tangible item where there is originally none (as in Dragulescu), or to highlight the way in which many elements composing viruses are manipulated and constructed to direct the viewer's perception of a certain entity (Jerram).

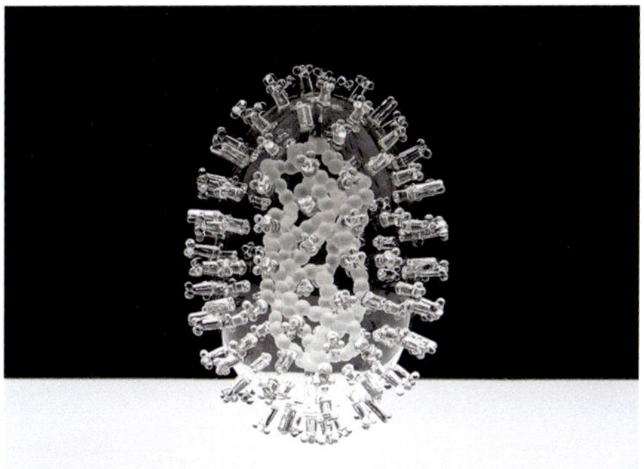

FIGURE 6 Avian Flu, *Glass Microbiology series. © Luke Jerram 2005.*

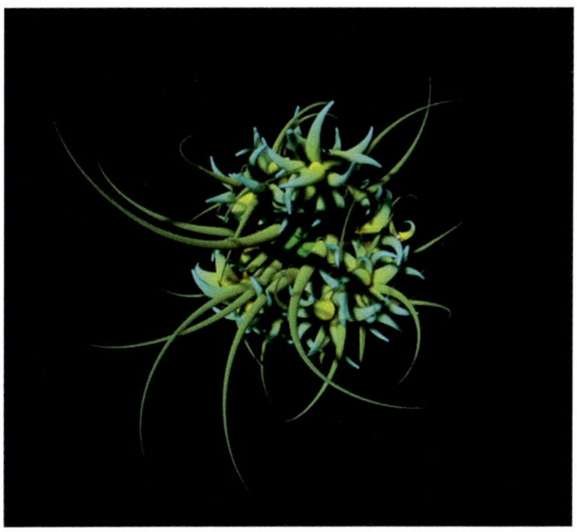

FIGURE 7 MyDoom, *Malwarez series. © Alex Dragulescu. 2008.*

Not only are the two images the product of different technical processes, but they also originate from two separate sets of knowledge. Jerram extracted the molecular model of N5N1 from the Protein Data Bank (PDB) and worked in collaboration with virologist Dr. Andrew Davidson from the University of Bristol to create a series of tangible, yet transparent, glass sculptures of (in)famous biological viruses and other potentially dangerous bacteria (Boustead 2009). The resulting series titled *Glass Microbiology* was created to emphasize the tension " … between the artworks' beauty and what they represent" and raised questions about how " … the coloring of scientific microbiological imagery affects our understanding of these phenomena" (Jerram 2018). Dragulescu has created a 3D rendering extracted from digitally native abstract data. The worm MyDoom—a resilient computer worm spreading via email and launching denial-of-service attacks (DoS) against CISCO and Microsoft environments—was commissioned by the security company MessageLabs. The company sent Dragulescu some previously neutralized codes of well-known viruses and worms (disassembled code, API calls, memory addresses and subroutines). Dragulescu used "algorithms to find recurring patterns in the source code of viruses and Trojans and then fed the results into a visualization algorithm" (Singel 2008). The artist admits to adding color-coding himself, with the rest of the image being generated by the data processed by the software.

I would like to draw attention on the ways the use of techniques of representations and choice of colors reveal specific cultural convergences. A first observation of the layout and presentation of these artworks (the classic portrayal of the virus emerging from a void and surrounded by nothing observed in the previous chapter) may suggest that a certain relatedness exists between the two objects, even though they never share the same ground. In fact, the first spreads among organisms while the second exclusively affects information networks. The two categories of viruses belong to different domains: carbon-based life and information.

Malware is often described as if it was a digital version of a corresponding biological threat. However, the actual physical intertwining of the two systems is still confined to the domain of science fiction, and in such texts this intertwining usually leads to rather odd consequences, as Bear's *Blood Music* demonstrated. In real life, the two realms are materially different. However, when it comes to building models for research or outreach purposes, examining the distinct material composition of biological and informational viruses, or researching and solving problems caused by them, biology and information become often interchangeable.

This occurs for a variety of reasons. The kinship existing between information and biological viruses is simultaneously metaphorical, cultural, material, and technical. First, whether we examine biological or informational threats, the instruments we use speak the same digital language. In fact, even biological viruses, when observed under a microscope, are immediately translated into digital format to be viewed on a screen, and readied to be colorized and enhanced digitally. Second, as it is visible from the images above, the way the two artifacts are displayed reveals many similarities, as if the two viruses belonged to the same realm: they are both portrayed in isolation from their surroundings, and their spherical and elliptical shapes are modeled as (biological and informational) virions, that is, in the form the virus molecule takes when is found intact, before it merges with its host. The similarities of the two images suggest an acknowledgment of their relationship (metaphorical or material), and an overall respect for certain stylistic conventions. As Bardini has suggested, such common visualizations offer a strategy to cope, a way to turn the unfamiliar into the familiar in order to comprehend it or to make it more acceptable.

Jerram and Dragulescu's artifacts are products of stylistic choices that reproduce viruses according to conventional and recognizable qualities. In fact, they convey a reading of viruses that feels consistent and suggests interesting similarities stemming from the geometric shapes used and the simplifications employed to produce images as plausible reproductions of viruses.

But what makes these two artifacts stand out from other typical representations of viruses is the presence of a couple of modifications. First, Luke Jerram's sculptures are transparent. As Kalliopi Monoyios observed upon visiting Jerram's collection of glass-blown microbiology sculptures, "something is captured in these sculptures that is lost in the false-color scanning electron microscope images we typically see of viruses and other extremely small subjects—the frailty of life, the beauty in vulnerability" (Monoyios 2013). In fact, microbiology models like the one we can freely download from the Protein Data Bank or the one we admire in science magazines and journals are typically artificially colored. Color choices and the use of geometrical contours are crucial in the interpretation of virus illustrations. For instance, personal or popular assumptions are confirmed and narratives are accepted when the application of technical procedures matches visual expectations. Although colors are often used for practical reasons—for example, the use of contrasting shades to distinguish between different parts—it becomes virtually impossible to distinguish how the elements emanating from popular narratives and those dictated by scientific and technical needs work together. Together, these elements both enable the immediate identification of viruses and simultaneously confirm the myths that surround viruses.

Making the virus transparent as well as shaping it as a solid sculpture invites reflections on the arbitrary application of colors in the representations of submicroscopic entities and its effects on entities widely regarded as dangerous. As an image, the virus becomes a colorless version of what we are generally used to see in magazines and journals. The contrast between the vividly colorful models gracing the covers of journals or included in science magazines and this colorless artifact invites reflections on the decisions made during the processes of visualizing and colorizing. Seeing the sculpture live allows the observer to seize the virus in its three dimensionality. Once the colors are gone, it becomes impossible for any viewer, even a relatively experienced one, to distinguish the many parts of the virus. This strategy also underlines the extent to which visualization practices reflect and, in turn, "adversely distorts the opinion of the viewer" (Boustead 2009), by manipulating their perception of the virus, even if this is done inadvertently.

Dragulescu's visualization of MyDoom is a speculative piece. Computer viruses and worms are not invisible because they are submicroscopic, but because they are made of data. They are purely abstract entities. Dragulescu took advantage of the unspecified conceptual and material exchanges between computer and biological viruses, modeling his visualization after one of the many typical molecular renditions of the viruses in circulation. Interestingly, all of the renditions in the series contain stylistic elements that simultaneously associate them with, and set them apart from their biological kin, making them distinctive yet correlated entities, as their content is made of data, not RNA, DNA, and proteins, and their natural environment is the information network and not biology. MyDoom may remind the viewer of familiar viruses such as HIV or RNA viruses such as coronavirus, whose spikes he elongated to reflect the data available, to convey more dynamicity, and to differentiate the computer worm from the biological viruses he drew upon. The virus also slightly resembles the biohazard symbol—with its spiky tentacles that allude to stingers, pincers, and danger. Dragulescu's image reveals how specific iconography originally used in biology has found its way into the realm of information. This strategy of visualization successfully establishes several cross-references between the realm of biology and the realm of information.

Stylistic and Methodological Crossovers

The comparison of computer systems to biological systems rendered in visual language by Dragulescu is neither surprising nor new. In a 1997 article published in the *Medical Journal of Australia*, we read: "Given their name, computer viruses are analogous to biological viruses, and analogies can be drawn between them in the prevention, detection, and treatment of infection" (Cheong and Kidd 1997, 45). In a similar way, Kephart, White, and Chess argue: "Biologists have combined the micro—and macroscopic perspectives on disease to good effect. It turns out that biological diseases and computer viruses spread in closely analogous ways, so that each field can benefit from the insights of the other" (Kephart, White, and Chess 1993, 22).

These statements indicate that the analogy between computer and biological viruses is based as much on assumed and intuitive elements as on (statistically) verified facts. The tendency to draw parallels between biological and informational viruses appears to be driven by similar understandings about their spread and their structure, and by a realization of the potential practical benefits that this comparison may achieve. Thanks to the scientific practice of using simple models to visualize complex concepts, the practice of "reduction" (Stengers 2010), similarities in structural and behavioral patterns can be easily compared across domains. Biology has come to borrow methodologies and instruments from information sciences while information sciences utilize immunological models deriving from the biomedical sciences to find new solutions to manage the ever-increasing number of threats being disseminated across digital networks. The same can be assumed when it comes to methods to detect, study, and neutralize viruses belonging to different realms.

Scientists and computer analysts applying these methods know well the issues and limitations associated with this practice. Nonetheless, they seem to be comfortable to integrate the terminologies of computer malware and biological agents. Scientific terms and methods have often become interchangeable across disciplines, confirming basic affinities. But the constant comparison leads to an almost automatic, if carefree, identification of a range of digital viral entities with biological entities and the assumption that the two environments that contain them share similar nature and functioning.

The persistent use of approximate terms to describe the features of viral entities indicates that an attempt is being made to both negotiate and take advantage of the complicated nature of viruses. As mentioned in the previous chapter, viruses have a peculiar nature that makes them hard to identify as self-contained and as predictable entities. This has to do with an industry and a research tradition that prefer determination and definition over elusiveness and indeterminacy. Thus, the very nature of viruses pulls the researcher between two poles: one that tries to define viruses as specific/defined entities, and the other that can't locate, and thus, can't escape, their aleatory nature: the ambiguous results seem to both satisfy and thwart both poles.

Biological viruses are said to have a "code," just like their computer peers have a "computer immune system" (Cheong and Kidd 1997). The exchange between information technologies and the life sciences becomes circular. This correspondence extends beyond terminology exchanges, appropriating and adapting entire methodological systems and strategies. "Nature has crafty ways to solve problems," Fernandes et al. write. For this reason, it has been a valuable inspiration for computer scientists throughout the years, as they attempt to "derive solutions for problems that may be otherwise hard or impossible to solve with other methods, possibly having higher computational complexity" (Fernandes et al. 2017). In fact, nature-inspired algorithms "abstract the phenomena found in the wild and are subject to evolutionary steps or computing layers in order to converge to a solution" (ibid.).

By comparing the complexity of the human immune system to the more discrete morphology of network systems " ... for detecting, identifying, and destroying most alien intruders" (Skormin et al. 2001), computer scientists have adopted approaches that are principally designed for the life sciences to study and strengthen "information security within an heterogeneous network of computers" (Villarreal 2005). In a chart where the comparison between biological and computer systems is fleshed out quite literally, Skormin et al. conclude that the two have stunning similarities: for example, the "alien microorganisms and malicious codes" they have to face are "composed of the same building blocks (basic amino acids and basic macro commands)"; similarly, as the "difference between alien microorganisms and the healthy cells of a biological system is in the (gene) sequencing of their building blocks," "the difference between malicious codes and the operational software of a computer network is in the sequences of their building blocks" (Skormin et al. 2001).

The popular view of the immune system that describes it as a citadel under attack by some pernicious enemy (Martin 1994) is linked to a sustained use of war metaphors. In Li and Knickerbocker's words, "both [computer and biological viruses] focus on subverting complex systems through weaknesses in design or environment" (J. Li and Knickerbocker 2007, 339). With the rise of malware, this citadel or complex system, like the immune system, is threatened by all sorts of attacks in the form of malicious code.

Table 1. Similarities Between Biological and Computer Systems

Biological Systems	**Computer Networks**
High complexity, high connectivity, extensive interaction between components, numerous entry points.	*High complexity, high connectivity, extensive interaction between components, numerous entry points.*
Vulnerability to intentionally or unintentionally introduced alien microorganisms that can quickly contaminate the system resulting in its performance degradation and collapse.	*Vulnerability to malicious codes (including computer viruses) that being introduced in the system result in unauthorized access to information and services and/or denial of service.*
Alien microorganisms as well as cells of a biological system are composed of the same building blocks - basic amino acids.	*Malicious codes as well as the operational software of a com puter network are composed of the same building blocks - basic macro commands.*
The difference between alien microorganisms and the healthy cells of a biological system is in the (gene) sequencing of their building blocks.	*The difference between malicious codes and the operational software of a computer network is in the sequencing of their building blocks.*
Biological immune systems ***are capable of*** *detecting, recognizing and neutralizing most alien microorganisms in a biological system.*	*Information security systems* ***should be capable of*** *detecting, recognizing and neutralizing most attacks on a computer network.*

FIGURE 8 *Table showing the similarities between biological and computer systems from an article in BASIS (Biological Approach to System Information Security). © Skormin et al. 2001.*

In the mid-1990s, Forrest, Hofmeyr, and Somayaji (1997) introduced an early computer immunology model based on the idea that the role of any immune system is to protect against intrusion by outsiders. This model focuses on building an "artificial immune system to protect computer networks based on immunological principles" (Hofmeyr and Forrest 2000) (its capacity to defend itself from internal and external attacks), and "algorithms and architecture" (445) (the immunology principle of negative selection). The computer immunology approach has become favored by those in security research seeking to understand the dynamics that regulate computer viruses and to produce antivirus software.

This engineering approach to immunology is particularly interesting, because of its ambition to propose a system that could be recirculated back into the biological sciences. Forrest claims that this approach could be potentially used to understand, if only partially, the functioning of all complex systems, including the immune system of a carbon-based organism. In considering how this might be done, Forrest asks several important questions: "[I]f we set out to engineer a protective system that operates successfully in an environment with some of the same constraints as those faced by the immune system, what components would we need and what would we need them for? To what extent would these components resemble the natural immune system?" (Forrest and Beauchemin 2007, 177).

The theorization and construction of what computer scientists call Artificial Immune Systems (AISs) constitute another example of the extent to which biological systems have been used as a model in computing. Using the affinities between biological systems and computer systems, an immunological approach for computers was devised using the model of a biological (modeled on a vertebrate organism, such as the mammals group) immune system. The operation of the latter was studied to discover how to identify network flaws in computer systems and build more efficient network security solutions. For instance, Dasgupta et al. describe the system devised by AIS as a "potential source of inspiration for novel approaches to solving complex computational problems, [as] its highly distributed, adaptive, and self-organizing nature, together with its learning, memory, feature extraction, and pattern recognition features offers rich metaphors for its artificial counterpart" (Dasgupta, Yu, and Nino 2011). AISs draw on the disciplines of immunology, computer science, and engineering, using metaphors (theoretical AIS), material applications (applied AIS), and mathematical models and simulations based on biological immune systems.

Computer security analysts have developed analysis and detection systems that identify and treat computer viruses and other malware in the same way an immunologist would treat biological trespassers.[1] In order to

[1]A detailed description of these projects can be found in Singh, P.K., and A. Lakhotia (2002). "Analysis and Detection of Computer Viruses and Worms: an Annotated Bibliography."

build better defenses against malware, they have meticulously compared biological systems to computer networks. BASIS (Biological Approach to System Information Security) was one of the first products of such research. Normally, Skormin observes, in order to be reliable, security systems have to process an enormous amount of data; this processing might slow down or negatively affect the functioning of the network. BASIS solves this problem by explicitly comparing and translating the principles that govern the immune system in a biological organism into a network context, creating "a number of semi-autonomous software agents to prevent particular kinds of threats and suppress specific types of attacks" (3), and recognizing and treating as a threat any illegitimate entry into the network system (Figure 8).

Artificial immune systems have been developed using theories drawn directly from the study of immunology. Initially relying on the concept of self *versus* non-self, that is, on the theory that an immune response is triggered when the body encounters something it designates as foreign, increasingly complex research on specialized AIS algorithms has acknowledged the importance of taking into consideration more nuanced theories, such as Polly Matzinger's "Danger Theory" (DT), in order to build more resilient and better responsive artificial immune systems. DT states that the immune system will only respond once it has already detected damage to cells, and not, as it was assumed before, when it detects specific antigen structures or bacterial products (a foreign body). As Matzinger explained in 1994 when her theory was first published, one would not explain why the human intestine does not react to, but instead hosts, entire colonies of bacteria that serve a symbiotic function, or why the immune system sometimes attacks its host as it does in the case of autoimmune diseases like multiple sclerosis and rheumatoid arthritis (Dreifus 1998; Matzinger 1994, 2012).

Fernandes et al. report that AISs are modeled in such a way that non-self is still neatly distinguished from self, the set characterizing normalcy in the system. Thus, AISs constitute a sort of compromise between the classic immunological theories, based on the central dogma of immunology, that is, self–non-self-discrimination, and the principles of clonal expansion and negative selection, which represent a more subtle position (Greensmith, Whitbrook, and Aickelin 2010)[2].

According to Chung-Ming Ou, Danger Theory here offers a more complex solution and becomes an efficient way to solve problems such as malware classification and anomaly detection. In fact, computer security systems in the form of antivirus software have "adopted some features inspired from the innate immune system, which can detect known malicious patterns. However, most commercial products do not yet have the capability

[2]Negative selection: T-cells and B-cells test for self-tolerance, that is, they are eliminated when they recognize self-molecules with high affinity. This process prevents the immune system from reacting against itself (general immune system) and to produce autoimmune reactions.

of adaptive immune system to address novel threats." To address this issue, "multiagent systems (MAS) provide the ability of distributed information security management" (Ou 2012). This model is more directly inspired from Matzinger's Danger Theory.

The decision to adopt an immunological model heavily depends on whether the model has been accepted by the immunological community, and while DT has gained a lot of traction in the recent years, it was, until recently, still considered by some a controversial theory (Aickelin and Cayzer 2002; Greensmith, Whitbrook, and Aickelin 2010). I would argue that the problem doesn't lie in the acceptance and adoption of the theory itself, but in the costs, the labor, and the CPU usage (or waste, depending on the user) that its adoption would mean for those building and using a commercial security system that is multilayered and contains enhanced numbers of variables. In fact, large corporations or government agencies might benefit from such system, because of the variety and frequency of threats they receive, and because of the size of the processors accommodating such system. However, home users might find such complex system superfluous or even cumbersome for the machines they operate.

Classifying and Representing as Culture

Ultimately, approximate descriptions, the reliance on metaphors and terms across disciplines to obtain meaningful comparisons, and the prolific cross-contamination of methods reflect both the difficulties involved in isolating and defining viruses and the often-arbitrary (and needed) decisions made in the analysis of their structure. In addition, these very descriptions and cross-contaminations help facilitate the dissemination of innovative approaches in computing security and immunology. The works presented in this chapter are exemplary. Jerram and Dragulescu's interpretations of biological and computer viruses condense the tensions between confining viruses to established categories and reproducing their vitality by producing images of similar design and layout; they make the circulation between biology and information visible by displaying different viruses using shared composition principles.

Unlike many of the images and the forms of representations of viruses being circulated, Jerram and Dragulescu's works introduce (or subtract) graphic elements that end up changing, thus suddenly making us aware of, the way we interpret viruses. In particular, Luke Jerram's glass sculptures of viruses' molecular sculptures expose issues regarding classification, by unmasking the politics behind the choices of color in visualization. Jerram observes that while color is clearly an artificially added feature for the microbiologist or the virologist, a non-scientist observer may wonder whether such coloring is reproducing the actual shades of the virus realistically (Jerram, n.d.). What color is a virus when it is found in nature? Jerram's colorless yet scientifically accurate three-dimensional models of deadly viruses not only raise this important question and lead to reflect on how decisions about colors are made, but also lay bare the rhetoric that accompanies the use of these—mostly bold, high contrast—colors, a rhetoric that stems from a cultural imaginary that associates them with fear and sickness.

In a similar way, Alex Dragulescu's visualization of the structures of a variety of computer viruses takes advantage of cultural references and paradigms adopted for the analysis of biological viruses. If we are willing to accept visualizations of computer viruses that are similar to those made for biological viruses, rather than imagining new ones that show the inherent features of computer viruses, then we also partially agree with these similarities. By using the stylistic elements that directly reference biological viruses, Dragulescu's visualizations of computer viruses accept and play along with the established parallelisms between information and biology, transmitting the same message to his viewer.

Jerram and Dragulescu's interpretations reproduce the issues that characterize the intersection between biology and information. For instance, the way viruses are located in—but don't really fit—traditional taxonomic categories, informs Jerram's and Dragulescu's artwork. While the reconstruction of the molecular morphology in Jerram's work and the illustration of code in Dragulescu's piece provide key for identification, they also transmit ideas that transcend biology and information. In the end, neither fully captures the real existence of the two entities. Something escapes explanation: it is impossible to tell to what extent this is an intentional omission or the product of a difficulty of expression, an arbitrary stylistic choice or the result of the acceptance of some stylistic obligations. This might be ascribed to the system of classification and taxonomy used.

The two interpretations expose the act of classifying, rendering, and representing as activities that are not solely technical or scientific, but also profoundly cultural. By manifesting as highly polished reproductions of provisional material; by providing a range of selected, yet sharply enhanced features only; by abiding by the model of the virus as isolated (or that can be potentially isolated) and as a loner, these artifacts confirm ideas of viruses that mostly bow to some established conventional rules. By explicitly appearing as digitally enhanced, or software manipulated entities, that is, as entities whose features overtly parade elements produced by human beings rather than as images of viruses as they allegedly naturally occur, they validate the invisibility of viruses. Despite the huge gap existing between informational and biological viruses, these artifacts are related, as they grow closer by virtue of their historically acquired and culturally suggested affinity.

The complexity of viruses, the difficulty involved in defining and representing them, is palpable in the way in which media and science amalgamate references to fiction and facts, and join art and science, even when the two are described as neatly separate. For instance, as news about infectious phenomena spread, top-down narratives and grassroots stories, rhetoric and personal accounts, scientific facts, and political interests become mixed. The boundaries between science and art, facts and rhetoric, scientific data recording and aesthetic appeal blur. This blurring, it must be noted, occurs in the scientific context as much as it does in the arts.

As Silvia Casini explains, "aesthetic qualities are already present in the laboratory," but "they remain hidden by the necessity of reading the image—data obtained according to the interpretative framework of the discipline performing the scientific operation" (Casini 2015). While elements inside the laboratory are already aesthetically charged, it is only in other contexts, outside of the lab, that their aesthetic potentials and their cultural significance become evident. For Casini, the context is determinant in activating other components: while these components are already present in images and other visual products generated by scientific processes, they may lie invisible when circulated within delimited disciplinary or technical circles.

This is important because images have been essential items for the transmission of knowledge since the rise of modern science; they are important tools, used to record experiments, to review findings, and to communicate them to external audiences—the virtual witnesses, who would be able to "see" or "imagine" and therefore reproduce such experiments mentally (Panese 2006). But in the context of science, functionality and pragmatism call for a variety of very specific narratives to obtain clarity, to convey certain meaningful findings or even simply to tell a story.

To be clear: visual renderings and theoretical models are culturally determined. Objects are "made observable" only when, and because, they serve specific functions. Hence, we find images of viruses as self-contained entities, we keep relying on simplified immunological models that may not work but they are convenient economically, make sense epistemologically, and can be easily communicated. Scientists often justify their choices of color, patterns, and structure, by invoking "pragmatism," arguing that the format of specific models or representations is dictated by the particular circumstances that produced the image, the audience targeted by said image, or the goals the scientist wishes to achieve—all items that involve aesthetic/artistic choices. This tendency is confirmed by many journals' recommendations for digital images: while image manipulation and enhancement are generally discouraged, "cleaning" visual noise and "sharpening" the image digitally in order to improve understanding are normally accepted and even considered more reliable (Frow 2014).

Along with the efforts of the scientific community to produce simple, acceptable models of viruses, it's important to note that individual interpretation need not conform to the expected response. Individuals, especially non-technical observers, who have trained eye to read a virus in the way a scientist or a designer meant to communicate, will decode scientific images according to their own outlooks, sometimes adding their contingent or personal interpretations.

Jerram's decision to omit colors in his series of glass models[3] significantly altered the way that observers perceive the significance of the pathogens standing in front of them. It made the politics of colored representations apparent to the uneducated spectator. On the other hand, Dragulescu's attempt to make a series of abstract bits of code visible revealed the difficult process of capturing, and later imagining, an entity that literally has no body. Here, conventional patterns were used to make the virus apparent.

It is precisely because of the work of artists and designers like Dragulescu and Jerram that the cultural and conventional significance of viral objects is made visible. Relocating these objects outside of the context in which they usually reside forces the observer to become more observant, to question the rationales behind the making of such models, to become aware of the "conventions and obligations" affecting the activity of scientists and other professionals, that is, the tensions existing between the necessity of the scientist to constantly catch up with an increasing variety of techniques, aesthetic experimentations, and the need to take into account disciplinary rules, industry customs, and public outreach requirements. When the two artworks are placed side by side, we also become increasingly aware of the continuity of information and biology both as two contexts naturally converging in the observation and description of objects and beings, as well as in the scientific analysis and investigation of complicated entities such as viruses.

[3]Luke Jerram's Glass Microscopy series is a collection of glass blown sculptures of popular viruses and bacteria's biomolecular models. His latest addition is, of course, SARS-CoV-2. "Made in glass, at 23cm in diameter" his website reads, "it is approximately 2 million times larger than the actual virus" (Jerram n.d; https://youtu.be/DdZBYKnSPeo).

3

Imagining Viruses

Seizing the Invisible: An Important Race

No matter how they are represented, viruses remain impossible to capture entirely by means of a single image. Motionless images and sculptural objects meant to depict the physical structure of biological viruses (or the idea of computer viruses), such as those created by Goodsell, Jerram, and Dragulescu, may convey a great sense of three-dimensionality, dynamicity, and scale but are still static artifacts. Their artworks capture an ephemeral moment—or a state, according to current virology (Cann 2012; Racaniello 2010; Wagner and Hewlett 2004), or a phase in a continuous process, as Dupré and Guttinger have come to define the life cycle of viruses (Dupré and Guttinger 2016)—of the existence of viruses.

The previous chapter examined visual artifacts to show how the difficulties involved in describing, defining, and visualizing viruses are both ontological (due to their nature) and epistemological (due to their qualities as products of the convergence of many socio-cultural vectors). This was evident in the ways viruses are named and incorporated into specific taxonomic groups, as well as in the way biology and information intersect and are called upon to better seize their morphology and behavior.

This chapter zooms in on the well-developed, yet relatively new art of visualization. Here, understanding the role of visualization as a process rather than a static product, and examining the way in which this process has been re-interpreted by artists takes center stage. As artist Tagny Duff argues, viruses are simultaneously "entity" and "movement," "living" and "undead," "material" and "dynamic" (Duff 2009). Jerram's glass models of popular viruses (Jerram, n.d.) described in the previous chapter pay tribute to the volatile matter of viruses, as well as to the conventional aesthetics that guarantee their acknowledgment as deadly viruses. His work displays the virus as a *virion*, the inactive state when the virus is still a virus particle or "spore" enclosed in its protective membrane (Racaniello 2020). This is also the most stable stage of viruses, one that can be well reproduced as a sculpture. It is also the most common, typical way in which viruses are visualized. Can all states and qualities of viruses be visualized, and visualized simultaneously? How can we seize each of their states, thus communicating their complex entanglement with the organic and the inorganic, the latter a legacy of the technologies and the modes of representation used?

With their composite, performative pieces, artists Caitlin Berrigan (Berrigan 2009) and Tagny Duff (Duff et al. 2011) demonstrate how viruses exceed the visual and structural constraints that science and conventional aesthetics have assigned to them. The two artists translate scientific facts and personal information into different media formats, the former through a series of chocolate sculptures faithfully shaped after the molecular model of hepatitis C retrieved from the Worldwide Protein Data Bank (PDB); the second, by indicating the presence of viruses using bio-markers "tattooed" on human and pig tissue. In both cases, viruses are inserted in a series of executions—rather than one sole image—that evoke the physical presence of the virus and its effects, its popular conception, and its existence and visual manifestation through technological instruments and laboratory processes.

Images assist us in comprehending the immaterial and the invisible: microscopic scans (used to examine virion morphology, structure, and dimensions, and presence or absence of an envelope), three-dimensional models (to highlight various aspects of the molecular composition of viruses), and other captivating illustrations for education and public consumption are only a few of the expressions competing to assign a visual appearance to viruses. This variety speaks to the current state of the scientific visualization of viruses; it both expresses the volatility of their nature and the determination to make these entities clear, discrete, and controllable. Importantly, it reveals what I see as a smooth dance between technical imagery and aesthetics: this dance is elegantly revealed through the many versions produced and published displaying the same virus, and the many aesthetic choices (through color, shapes, layout, etc.) made when a virus is analyzed and explained. As a matter of fact, the debate on whether to erase aesthetics from scientific images, thus reducing the visualization to a mere technical illustration, has a long history.

Despite the sophisticated methods available today, the size and nature of viruses make finding a single appropriate visualization model and method of analysis challenging. Viruses have no immediately visible body—biological viruses are so small that a light microscope is often not sufficient to capture their shapes, and computer viruses have no tangible material shape at all. A particularly complicated process leads to the visualization of biological viruses: electron microscopes and customized software are used to capture viruses by subjecting them to technological and chemical processes before they reach the covers of journals and magazines. These instruments are used to obtain temporary impressions of a virus's appearance, generating provisionary, as well as highly customized images. The lack of data, or, paradoxically, the overabundance of data extracted from these submicroscopic entities, as well as the lengthy and laborious processes applied to isolate and immortalize them end up further complicating, not simplifying the operation of visualization. As a result, visual renderings and illustrations become the product of multiple stages of data analysis, parts selection, as well as conceptual and visual interpretation.

The elusiveness and the perceived disruptive qualities of viruses generate expectations affecting the way scientists, technicians, or graphic designers (the producers of images) and the public (the consumers of images) approach them, and construct (or appreciate) their visual representations. The interest in computer and biological viruses, both among scientists and the public, has contributed to the creation of more ways of illustrating them, adding to the already considerable variety of visual renditions. Scientific research focusing on biological viruses has produced more and more refined visualizations by employing the growing repertoire of technological devices available, and by exploiting their cultural interpretations. Because of the cultural references these illustrations contain, they are appreciated by the professional as well as by a far less scientifically literate and diverse public.

In the case of computer viruses, the path toward visualization takes a different trajectory. In fact, creating a visual rendition of Malware is certainly not the principal priority of the computer science community. Images of computer viruses like Dragulescu's are often made as special art commissions that rarely contribute to research on computer virus threats. This is in part due to the goals and the commercial nature of the sector conducting the study of viruses: computer virus researchers and security analysts primarily work for companies specialized in creating antivirus software. In these companies, understanding how malware works is mainly directed at finding vulnerabilities. Security systems are then built with these vulnerabilities in mind. Thus, the most common form of visualization is the one that inserts the virus in a map, favoring its epidemiological behavior rather than its morphology, since the focus is on the process of infection, not on the virus per se. When visualization happens, computer viruses display visual patterns that, on the one hand, directly connect them to their biological relatives, reproducing similar aesthetics and forms. On the other hand, they provide novel ways to look at viruses by using animations and by imagining visualization techniques able to render their dynamic movement through networks and operating systems.

Because of the difficult processes leading to the visualization of biological viruses, and the radically different paths and preferences chosen by the computing sector, this chapter will leave malware behind for now. As it will be clear in next chapter, the cross-pollination of information and biology in the treatment of viral phenomena continues and intensifies when viruses are studied from an epidemiological angle, as mathematics and data visualization via big data engage in a fascinating exchange across the two domains.

One and Many

Given the specialized resources and methods utilized to study viruses, their visual renderings are unsurprisingly numerous, giving the impression that there are no fixed or established rules that apply to the visualization of viral material. However, the diversity of visualization is not the result of arbitrary decisions. Visualization is mostly the product of lab and data retrieval protocols and frequently conforms to recognizable visual tropes and aesthetic preferences. For example, in the previous chapters, both David Goodsell and Luke Jerram made substantial use of the molecular data of the Protein Data Bank (PDB). The use of this and other online protein databases contributes to partially homogenize the basic models used for the illustrations. But this still leaves a great deal of variety. In fact, different models are often produced by different labs: they exhibit variations, privilege certain sets of data over others, and make different choices regarding colors, according to the goal of the model. When displayed as illustrations, or as animated sequences, viruses retain only very basic characteristics of the microscopic scans and scientific models originally used to generate them: variety and heterogeneity abound, as viruses are not simply reproduced, but also imagined. The information extracted from protein databases serves only as a starting point. It undergoes several transformations, in the hands of individual scientists and scientific teams, software applications and graphic designers; it is customized and adapted to different circumstances and types of publications.

The scientific visualization of viruses contains a tension between two contending forces. The first seeks to implement a clear model that incorporates normative rules and retains basic cultural references. The second seeks to escape them. These competing forces are at play in every stage of the visualization process, including those stages involving the producers of the visualizations (laboratories, graphic studios), and the consumers (other scientists and different audiences with different levels of media literacy). It is only by keeping in mind all stages of the process of visualization that one can truly appreciate the complex socio-technical articulation and the concerted role played by laboratories, graphic studios, and the public in contributing to the final image.

Acknowledging the constructed nature of viral representations and the competing forces at play in the creation of those representations generates questions about their role, and specifically, about the extent to which arbitrary and instrumentalizing aesthetics, scientific and technical limitations are involved in the realization of these images. A quick web search of "visualization of viruses" brings up a great number of different images. In some cases, the results will reveal many versions of the same virus, sporting different colors, with more or less enhanced forms and geometric shapes. Science Librarian Erik Svallingson, for instance, observed the following about the plethora of images that have been circulating about the SARS-CoV-2 viruses: "These images seem intended to capture the reader's interest, but are also clearly variations on a theme: strong colors and obviously exaggerated shapes that enhance the virus's spiky, club-like appearance" (Svallingson 2020). All of this fosters the impression that viruses are so elusive that no clear, definite picture can be produced. It also raises suspicion about the scope and the intentions behind these images: even when made with good intentions, visual communication scholar Colette Gaiter argues, images displaying high contrast colors, or enhanced and overly emphasized geometry, especially when they are disseminated during a crisis (like during the SARS-CoV-2 pandemic) risk quickly becoming "a simplified representation that people instantly recognize—and a symbol for the terrifying and wildly contagious virus that has put the world on hold" (Gaiter 2020). Producing a visualized rendition of a virus is a balancing act as it passes through technical, cultural, and political filters.

To a degree, variety is the direct result of the elusive nature of viruses. The urge to produce discrete knowledge out of the ambiguity manifested by the subject reproduced can be traced historically, when the separation between technical forms of representation and added aesthetics was consolidated. Stemming from the notion that seeing is a form of knowing, the technical image is assumed to quantify and provide an image of the object unspoiled by distracting aesthetics. This idea of objectivity, as Daston and Galison explained in Chapter 2, historically started with the Scientific Revolution, has taken many forms, with the main challenge being how to exclude the presence of the "subjective" human from the scientific object. The tendency to think of knowledge in terms of the ability to delimit and measure an object reflects the assumption that representation plays a mere mediating role between the knower and the known, the observer and the observed (Barad 2007). While this representationalist approach has been generally disproved, it is very much still alive in the visualization of viruses. In fact, despite being well-aware that any visual rendition produced will stand as a placeholder of the entity, scientists and graphic designers prefer not to implement ways of rendering and modes of representation that are completely novel or unique. Visual innovation is to be found in incremental improvement rather than in the imagination of completely new modes of display, with the use of new technologies and instruments with increasingly high resolution, as well as the mastery of a combination of software and selective research to track and display a virus.

Two important recent examples from early (but constantly updated) attempts to render the molecular composition of the SARS-CoV-2 virus are cases in point. The first (Figure 9) is the now iconic red and white model created in February 2020 by Alissa Eckert and Dan Higgins for the Centers for Disease Control and Prevention (CDC 2020); the second (Figure 10) is Veronica Falconieri Hays's 3D model of the virus produced for the July 2020 special issue of *Scientific American* (Falconieri Hays 2020). When observed side by side, the two models show that in each case the form and parts of the coronavirus have been partly inferred from existing models (the first SARS virus being an important start [Figure 11A and B]), selected from different research labs, or arbitrarily determined (the choice to display or not display a stem in the spikes, the choice of colors [Figure 11C]). These images are both technically and technologically innovative, clearly carrying the aesthetic signature of the authors. However, the authors chose not to distance themselves from the current visual conventions, delivering visualizations that could be easily read.

As Barad explains,

> Liberal social theories and theories of scientific knowledge alike owe much to the idea that the world is composed of individuals—presumed to exist before the law, or the discovery of the law—awaiting/inviting representation. The idea that beings exist as individuals with inherent attributes, anterior to their representation, is a metaphysical presupposition that underlies the belief in political, linguistic, and epistemological forms of representationalism.
>
> (Barad 2007)

In its attempt to render this or that aspect of viruses resulting in a great variety of visual renderings, scientific visualization refutes the myth that there exists a pristine "natural" and distinct pure entity hidden somewhere (be it made of information or made of biology), a "thing in itself" waiting to be represented. In fact, the processes of data retrieval and art of display demonstrate how the "thing" called virus cannot become visible, unless it is subjected to chemical processes, technological transcoding, design protocols, all of which involve the ambition and creative input of individuals engaged in the visualization business.

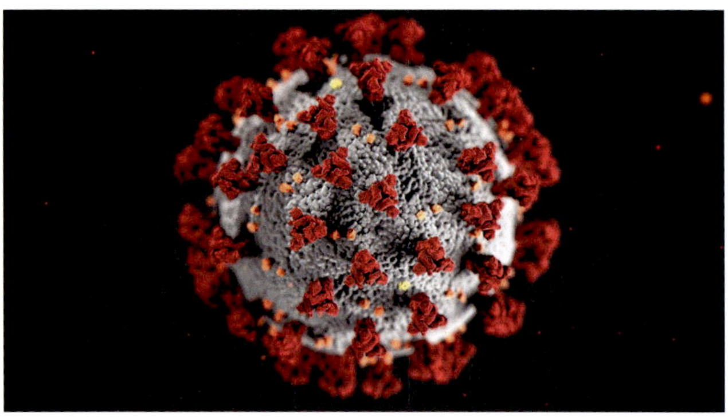

FIGURE 9 *Alissa Eckert and Dan Higgins' model for the Centers for Disease Control and Prevention (CDC).* https://phil.cdc.gov/Details.aspx?pid=23311

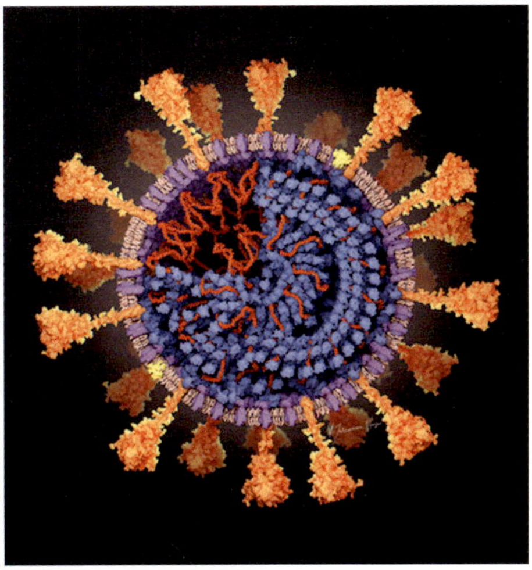

FIGURE 10 *SARS-CoV-2 in 3D. 3D model of the virus produced for the July 2020 special issue of* Scientific American. © *Veronica Falconieri Hays.* https://www.scientificamerican.com/author/veronica-falconieri-hays/

Visualization, Bìos, and Politics

Thanks to scientific processes (e.g., electron microscopy) and visualization strategies (e.g., visualization software), viruses can be turned into visual artifacts for public consumption. Molecular models, microscopy scans, and other colorful images visually rendering specific viruses grace the pages of popular science magazines and peer-reviewed journals. There is a general tendency to largely accept these images as products derived from direct scrutiny of viruses by means of high-resolution devices (Pauwels 2006, viii): in fact, increasingly higher resolution and technological innovation are often the two most emphasized qualities when a new image of a virus is being disseminated publicly.

The emphasis on technology and innovation has been particularly strong during the SARS-CoV-2 pandemic as several labs shared resources and technologies to co-produce models and illustrations using the most recent findings about the virus. The focus on detailed, high-resolution images of the virus produced by state-of-the-art software could be observed in the images above and in well-curated articles where viruses are analyzed in all their parts, expertly colorized, animated, and inserted into dynamically designed web essays (Corum and Zimmer 2020; Sarkar 2021; Zimmer 2020). In front of the parade of colorfully rendered illustrations of viruses, vis-à-vis the emphasis on resolution and magnification that accompany them, audiences at all levels of visual literacy and scientific knowledge may be easily made to assume that what appear in the pages of those magazines are magnified reproductions of viruses.

If we were to peel off the layers building one of those images, we would probably find the remnants of a microscopic scan. The scan is what is accepted to be the virus, or rather the virion standing for the virus surrounded by a protective capsid. The scan is an entry point into the visual reconstruction of the virus: in fact, in cases of novel viruses, such as the current coronavirus, viruses belonging to the same family—not the specific virus—were used as starting point (Christiansen et al. 2020; Falconieri Hays 2020).

Obtaining an electron microscope scan is neither easy nor straightforward: the first scan was not produced until the first half of the twentieth century, thanks to the invention of the electron microscope. In 1932, Max Knoll and Ernst Ruska, German physicists, successfully built a prototype transmission electron microscope (TEM), which subsequently was perfected by a team of scientists at the University of Toronto (Prebus 1998; Rasmussen 1996).

The TEM was a major breakthrough in microscopy. Unlike light microscopes that operate by diffracting light and which have relatively limited resolve power, electron microscopes use beams of electrons whose wavelength is over 100,000 times shorter than visible light photons. This enables levels of magnification that are millions of times stronger than those obtained with light microscopes (Goldsmith and Miller 2009). Today, many viruses are captured thanks to cryoEM microscopes. Here, in addition to using electrons, the specimen is subjected to very low temperatures in order to achieve better resolution. Currently, these are considered some of the most powerful microscopes in circulation, often predilected by illustrators and visual communicators (Earl et al. 2017).

Electron microscopes with such augmented capacity are neither user-friendly nor cost-effective instruments, and the operations required to capture the molecular content of viruses are quite labor-intensive (Flegler, Jr, and Klomparens 1997; L. P. Villarreal 2005). First, these microscopes require a dedicated environment as well as trained personnel to configure and calibrate the instrument and to operate its software (Goldsmith and Miller 2009; University of Cambridge 2012). Second, prior to exposing a virus specimen to the electron beams of a TEM and cryoEM, or a scanning electron microscope (SEM), a multi-phase preparation is required. Biological specimens need to be prepared (i.e., protected and preserved) by means of fast freezing, using liquid nitrogen for the former or staining and coating the sample with the heavy metal osmium for the latter (Chandler and Roberson 2009). Importantly, because the instrument works by directing electrons onto the specimen, it needs to operate in a vacuum. Scientists supervise the process and prepare the specimen by applying exact amounts and proportions of chemicals and minerals so as to not compromise the sample's integrity. Third, since these procedures are performed on very small-scale objects, they are prone to both errors and safety hazards (e.g., exposure to damaging agents) (Berge 1999). Thus, the success of this process depends on a variety of skills and calls for the intervention of a range of well-trained individuals.

Once samples of viruses are selected, stained, or frozen, other procedures are conducted to further dissect and examine their anatomy. The visual product obtained from the electron microscope appears as a black-and-white image displaying a conglomerate of viruses. Its resolution varies according to the preparation technique, the goal established by the investigators, and the state of the microscope (Chandler & Roberson 2009). In the meantime, the image extracted from the sample has already gone through a process of digitization, and it is now ready to be analyzed, colorized, enhanced, and turned into one of the many images we see circulating (Figure 11A, B and C).

The processes viruses undergo in the lab and the following work done to present them in a readable visual format unavoidably produce a variety of differently processed and designed images. This material heterogeneity in no way can provide a standardized imagery. To explain how these seemingly contradictory aspects coexist, I am drawn to Roberto Esposito's analysis of the two Foucauldian concepts of biopower and biopolitics: "In what sense does life govern politics, or in what sense does politics govern life? Does it concern the governing of or over life?" (Esposito 2008, 15). To put those questions in the context of scientific visualization, this may translate as: in what way are these visual renditions of viruses the product of a series of established conventions, cultural beliefs, and instrumentalizations (biopower, or governance as the subjection of life to politics)? And in what way do we construct visualization to adapt to the changing notion of viruses or to the different views we can obtain from their different statuses (biopolitics, when we construct politics in the name of life)?

To identify the role of these two forces at play in the scientific visualization of viruses, centering one's examination on the sole published image is not sufficient. Acknowledging the processes and the socio-political dynamics that have produced them may shed some light on the many vectors contributing to such operation.

As Natasha Myers (2014) suggests, the act of visualizing as an act of rendering is not just a matter of reproducing an "object that can stand in for something else," it is also a combination of gestures, performative by nature, referring not just to "the object that is rendered, but also to the subject, the one who renders, and the activity of rendering" to "pass an object or

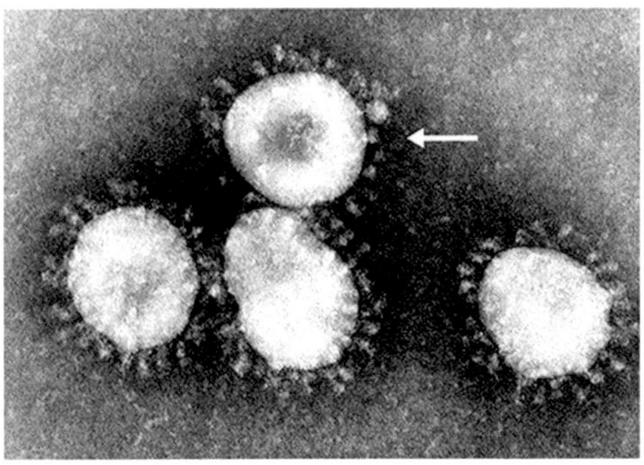

FIGURE 11A *Electron microscopy image of SARS-CoV, with the arrow pointing at a single virion. Several early visualizations of SARS-CoV-2 used these early 2000s pictures as basis. Photo: Dr. Fred Murphy. Courtesy the Centers for Disease Control and Prevention's (CDC) Public Health Image Library (PHIL), identification number 4814 (https://phil.cdc.gov/Details.aspx?pid=15523).*

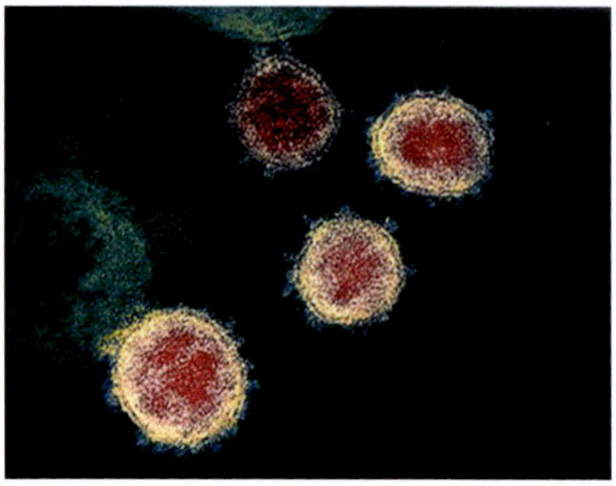

FIGURE 11B *Transmission electron microscope image shows SARS-CoV-2, the virus that causes COVID-19, isolated from a patient in the United States. Virus particles are emerging from the surface of cells cultured in the lab.*

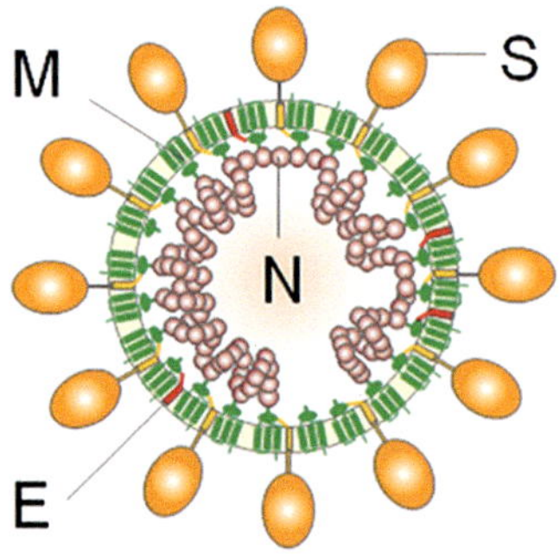

FIGURE 11C *Schematic diagram of coronavirus virions.*

communication from one person to another" (Myers 2014, 154). Rendering involves not just the production of an object that stands in for something else (i.e., the creation of an image to represent a virus), it also involves a combination of gestures that she defines as being "performative" by nature. The complexity of the phenomena resulting from the data-mining process is selectively "curated" to give space to consistent results or to give rise to plausible and easily readable outcomes. Here, richness and diversity are tamed in favor of clarity. The reduction that is the product of digitization and visualization is a metaphoric necessity and not just an "aesthetic flourish" (Michael Lynch 1988, 159). The metaphors comprising this process are lures that direct practitioners' imaginations and experimental inquiry (Stengers 2010). Visualization then is "like the materialized refiguration that corporealize[s] life in the form of information systems" (Myers 2014, 142). Commenting on early visualizations created from data, McCormick observed how processes of visualization "transform the symbolic into the geometric" (McCormick 1988). The challenge of visualization is to "come up with a design metaphor that will accommodate the transformations from non-spatial, non-numerical concepts to something visible and meaningful" and will make sure that the "particular metaphor does, indeed, work" (Chen 2005, 29).

I would like to propose an analysis of the process that produces visualization, one that examines the way in which the historical practices of scientific illustration and the present context surrounding the creation of viral illustrations, the labor and the technological apparatus utilized, inform the nature of the images produced. All intersecting technical and scientific aspects of visualization, including expectations and tacit rules, shape and are shaped by the visual products emerging at the end of the process (Ruivenkamp and Rip 2014). "The laboratory," Coopmans (2014) explains, "extends to other spaces and places via collaborative ventures, shared data centres, and information and communication technologies," challenging "the very distinction between laboratory and field" (Coopmans 2014, 3). Inspired by Latour's (1983; 1988) actor network theory and Latour and Woolgar's (1979) analysis of the rich activity and relationships interwoven and performed in the laboratory, researchers have increasingly understood this space as composite and multilayered, containing a range of instruments, protocols, processes, and power relations (Latour 1988, 1979; Latour 1988; Latour and Woolgar 1979).

Typically, the exploration of viruses through specific instruments and given procedures aims at a clear definition of these entities as distinct scientific objects, an operation that Lynch calls a "domestication" (Lynch 2006). This is usually a collaborative endeavor. Several professionals and specialized labs are involved in the theorization and implementation of 3D models and scientific illustrations (Chandler and Roberson 2009). While the SARS-CoV-2 Atomistic model made by Nanographics GmbH mentioned in Chapter 1 is certainly a clear example of such collaborative effort ("Nanographics—Scientific Visualizations" n.d.), Eckert and Higgins, on the one hand, and Falconieri, on the other, had to combine a number of studies, existing models, and earlier research in order to complete their illustrations (Falconieri Hays 2020).

The nature of viruses and the different technologies and techniques used produce different results. In addition, scientists, lab technicians, and graphic designers are urged to develop innovative visualization techniques as part of the continuous quest for innovation. The resulting images reflect an aggressive historical and cultural notion of seeing as conquest, as manipulation, and colonization of the invisible (Virilio 2000). At the same time, visualization reflects a certain abhorrence of the "unseen" and the "undetermined," as if they were threats to be put under control. Visualization then becomes a form of control over what appears to be difficult to control.

Today's expanding area of visualization tends to abide by a double biopolitical paradigm. Foucault defined biopower as the most recent power configuration in a three-stage system: a sovereign and juridical power, a power based on "disciplinary mechanisms," and a system whose "purpose is not to modify any given phenomenon as such, or to modify a given individual insofar as he is an individual, but, essentially, to intervene at the level at which these general phenomena are determined, to intervene at the level of their generality"(Foucault 2003, 245). This regime of power brings neither substantial nor revolutionary changes to the current system, but it makes sure that the system maintains a balance by anticipating any surprises. Unlike sovereignty or the power to "take life and let live," to decide whether to let people live or die, biopower is the "power to intervene to make live," that is, to regulate the life of those who are alive (Foucault 2008). Biopower seeks to achieve a mastery at the level of life itself (Macey 2009), "taking control of life and the biological processes of man-as-species and of ensuring that they are not disciplined, but regularized" (Foucault 2003, 246).

The notion of "population," Foucault reminds us, replaces the one of "individual," that is, the heterogeneous group comprising of distinct elements (the individuals) is gradually reduced to "a mass of living and coexisting beings," a non-descript and anonymous agglomerate of discrete components, its collective behavior measured and quantified with the purpose of preventing, not correcting or isolating, unexpected episodes or dramatic changes (like the incidence of diseases and epidemics, or the spread and the appearance of a virus). Mechanisms such as "forecasts, statistical estimates, and overall measures" are the new ways in which population is kept under control. The mechanisms introduced by biopower are not directly coercive, but operate by measuring general trends, mapping tendencies, extrapolating phenomena, and, ultimately, by releasing recommendations on the way the population ought to behave in order to mitigate unexpected episodes of disruption of the system. The anomaly and the unexpected are brushed away by identifying them before they occur and by subsequently finding ways to prevent them from emerging or to limit their impact.

Biopower permeates the practice of visualization, when it embodies a mechanism comparable to the way forecasts and statistics act upon the population. It does so by capturing molecular structures by means of estimates and approximations (by evincing shapes and structures from scans that are difficult to read and complex chemical configurations); or by seizing their typical and average characteristics, rather than their single behaviors and unique structures (by downloading and comparing different molecular models from the PDB). For example, Veronica Falconieri explains how in creating a 3D model of the SARS-CoV-2 virus, she had decided to combine new data and data deriving from EM scans of SARS-CoV. In fact, although the two viruses are distinct, they share over 90 percent of their physical and genomic qualities and have a very similar appearance. To this as a starting point, she added new data from the Amaro Lab at the University of California San Diego (Falconieri Hays 2020).

Parallels can be drawn between the way in which Foucault (2007) describes the relation between security and population and the relation that exists between visualization and viruses. Like security, whose aim is to study a phenomenon in order to anticipate its behavior and minimize any adverse surprise it may cause (Thacker 2009; Foucault, 2008; van Loon 2002a; 2002b), visualization monitors and studies the structure, the development, and the mechanisms by which viruses spread, in order to seize—and later predict—their behavioral patterns.

Visualization is also tied to aesthetic and cultural norms. Given that, two complementary questions arise: Can scientific information about viruses be interpreted and/or discerned uniformly? How can predictions be made when the object of research is not a fixed one? With mutating objectives tied to different contingencies and institutional practices, and with software or personal choices in visualization, diversification is unavoidable. But here is where scientific visualization expresses complications pertaining to the governing of the life of viruses, and therefore to the biopolitics of visualization. First, it faces obligations to regulate the form and aesthetics of the illustrations disseminated (to make the virus recognizable, to abide by branding directives of labs and graphic studios, etc.). Second, it is confronted by an opposite push to innovate, transform, and modify the way in which they appear visually, not only because of the emphasis on technological innovation described earlier, but also because of a desire to propose new modes of representations. Because of these tensions, what is communicated is partial and simplified.

Visualization is also caught up in another biopolitical dilemma. According to Roberto Esposito's philosophical analysis of biopolitics, "the terms from which biopolitics is formed (life and politics) cannot be articulated except through a modality that simultaneously juxtaposes them" (Esposito 2008, 32). This gap is revealed through the encounters between the scientific investigations that visualization supports and viruses, whose aleatory nature (the submicroscopic size, the frequent mutations, the multi-state nature) obstructs attempts to obtain definite investigations. In other words, viruses cannot be fully tamed, or represented in fully novel ways. As Esposito explains, "Either life holds politics back, pinning it to its impassable natural limit, or, on the contrary, it is life that is captured and prey to a politics that strains to imprison its innovative potential." Biopolitics " … becomes the governance of vital forces" (Thacker 2009, 136), or the attempt to regulate something that cannot be regulated not only because of its own shifting nature, but also because of the forces and pressures that shape or modify it as well as the sheer amount (or the lack) of information collected and produced through the visualization process.

The proliferation and the variety of scientific visualization are one material manifestation of the power game between bìos (the vitality and the provisional nature of viruses) and politics (the material instruments, the historico-cultural harnesses, and the aesthetics). The Sisyphean exercise of upgrading visualization devices and imaging techniques reflects the desire to convey clarity. However, this striving inevitably contributes to diversification rather than standardization, or, better yet, diversification within partial standardization. At the same time, the drive to engage with virtually incessant innovation in visualization techniques and aesthetics becomes a delicate task of balancing the constraints, the fixed set of regulations imposed by institutions and publications, and the tropes and standards dictating how viruses must or should be represented. Finally, as advances in imaging technology have allowed the rendering of ever-smaller details, the picture of the viral object is enriched, and previously invisible details are further revealed. At the same time, the viral object inevitably drifts farther away, taking on an appearance that resembles less of a natural organism and more of a computer-generated being or an entity that could as well live in a computer (Robins and Webster 1999).

Entity and Movement: Performing Viruses

I have observed how visualization cannot contain in one image the different states through which viruses manifest, nor can it (and nor does it want to) simultaneously represent the different phases of preparations, digital manipulations, and reductions comprising the process of visualization. Even though it can be inferred that an illustration of a virus has undergone some manipulation, it is certainly impossible to tell what type and at what stage it has occurred.

I am reminded of Goodsell's two illustrations of the coronavirus: in order to show the different statuses of the virus, he had to create two distinct images, one as a virion, just before the virus attached itself to the host, and one during the process of infection, when the virus was already active. What if viruses were not made evident through two-dimensional imaging? What if different media or objects were able to convey the above states, what if they were able to flesh out their dynamicity? Could they function as alternative forms of visualization? Would they foster a better comprehension of the virus in all its multifaceted complexities, or would they evoke more questions about its nature and the hosts it affects?

Sitting nicely in a glass jar lie some chocolate truffles. These chocolate treats are molded after a magnified 3D cryo-electron micrograph of the hepatitis C virus (i.e., a cryo-EM model of the virion-sized capsid[1]), retrieved from the Protein Data Bank (PDB) (Figure 13). In *Viral Confections* (Figure 14), Caitlin Berrigan, at the time affected by hepatitis C, created the work to stir a discussion about what it means to carry a virus that affects around four to five million people in the United States alone. While the subject of the work may be repugnant (the virus is the cause of a disease that can result in severe illness and even death), the form of the work, chocolates wrapped in an elegant package and offered to visitors of the exhibition, is enticing.

Chocolate is a highly ductile material which tends to crumble and break when it's too dry, and to melt easily when the temperature rises. These qualities make chocolate an excellent material for the work. Chocolate stains and sticks, it may soften, leaving imprints and traces over any surface with which it comes in contact. This may provide an accurate, yet imperfect

[1]A capsid consists of a series of protein subunits coating the virion's nucleic acid. A capsid is one of the major criterions for the classification of viruses.

reproduction of the protein structure of the virus. It gives us, the viewers, a hint of the quick transfer that the virus molecule is capable of.

Berrigan's body of work related to the hepatitis C virus consists of several installations forming a formidable discussion piece. The artist has exhibited these both individually and as part of a more comprehensive corpus she entitled *Sentimental Objects in the Attempt to Befriend a Virus*. In addition to the chocolate truffles, this corpus consisted of a large-scale, three-dimensional rendition of the geodesic structure according to which the hepatitis C virus organizes its proteins (or capsid). This shelter was built during a Beam Camp in New Hampshire where Berrigan worked on a piece with the campers. The participants in the camp dressed the domes themselves, using tasteful golden fabric. This color is a reminder of the jaundice that hepatitis C causes in those affected by the disease. To the shelter, she added a letter to the virus, in which she provides facts and statistics on hepatitis C,

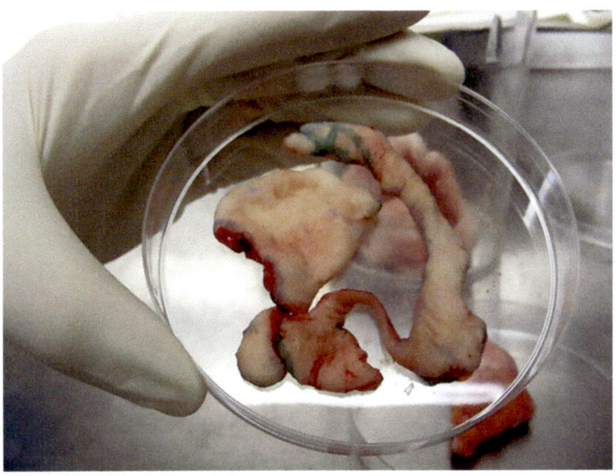

FIGURE 12 *Tagny Duff,* Living Viral Tattoos, *2009. Detail of pigs tissue stained by the virus spreading across the skin.*

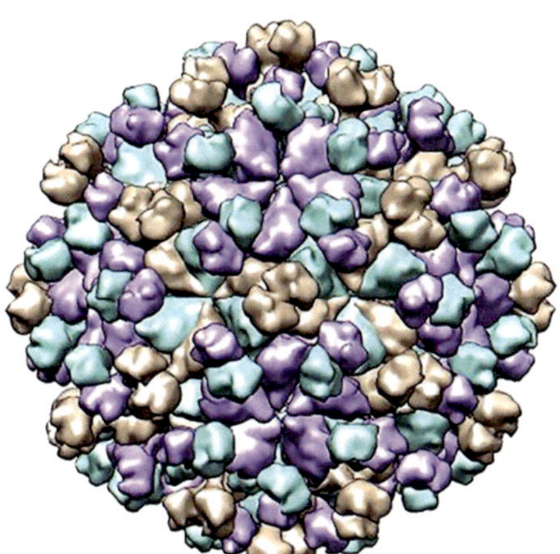

FIGURE 13 *The cryo-EM model used by Berrigan. This model can be created and downloaded from the PDB. Visualized using Jmol.*

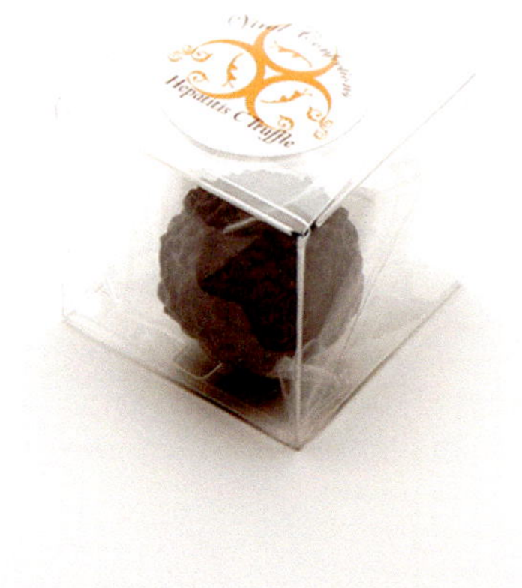

FIGURE 14 *Caitlin Berrigan,* Viral Confections. *Single wrapped chocolate candy bearing the form of the hepatitis C virus from PBD. © Caitlin Berrigan, 2006.*

addressing the virus as if it was a potential friendly companion. At a Gallery 400 exhibition in Chicago titled *Biological Agents* (October 2008), she welcomed the visitors inside this shelter-sized geodesic structure to consume the chocolate viruses and to engage in a conversation about the spread and effects of hepatitis C.

The scientific material used for the model, the epidemiological facts concerning the incidence of the virus, the conventional representations of its protein structure, and its assumed qualities are all displayed in the same exhibition. The processes and methods of visualization are made apparent in the creation of multiple different renderings of the same object-virus as a molecular model turned into a sculpture, a capsid taking the form of a geodesic shape, a booklet that functions as both an informational brochure and a love/hate note to the hepatitis C virus, an invisible entity living in the body of the artist and in who knows how many other individuals. This configuration reveals the diversity of forms that viruses can take each time their appearance is made evident; in turn, this helps in understanding how viruses can be perceived through images and visual models, as much as through other objects and constructions; finally, it produces new awareness of their mediated nature.

With its size magnified and its appearance multiplied (the candies and the shelter) and its materiality reproduced by different media (chocolate and fabric over wires, architectural structure, and edible treat), the virus materializes as a distributed entity whose boundaries exceed its conventional self-contained representation. In other words, from single, hepatitis C becomes multiple, its invisible presence is made visible not by means of a single artifact, but by way of a fluid world of objects and humans engaging in conversation about its materiality and liminality. From invisible threat, the virus turns into a tangible series of objects with which viewers can connect; its identity as threat temporarily dissipates, as the virus's protective shell becomes a shelter for the audience and its encounter with its host is re-dressed as a pleasant experience of chocolate tasting.

The various ways in which the virus is reproduced can be both enticing and revolting: the chocolate truffles are elaborate and delicious, yet they represent an infamous virus. The informative pamphlet containing important information on the infectious rates of the disease and on the symptoms that this disease causes is written in the very personal form of a love letter addressed to the virus. The audience might misunderstand the facts as fiction, or, conversely, might not appreciate or necessarily agree with the personal form of the document: this all comes down to the personal encounters and the personal experience of the different audiences with the virus. Importantly, the chocolate tasting exercise; the making of, and the welcoming dome; and the letter to the virus prompts a series of collective experiences. This contrasts with the often solitary journey the patient affected by hepatitis C is forced to face, because of the stigma it carries (Berrigan 2020).

Following different methodologies but using a similar conception of the virus as situated, Tagny Duff's *Living Viral Tattoos* reflects on its impermanent and dynamic nature through the performative practice of bioart (Figure 12). The virus, according to Duff, "as entity and event, transverses the threshold of living and undead. The virus is exemplary in that it proposes a complex threshold of liveness and exceeds it" (Duff 2009). Working with the lentivirus, a synthetic retrovirus, Duff explored "ideas of the viral through learning and applying biological synthetic viral vectors as both material and object of artistic creation" (37).

Viruses are scientifically defined as "living" or active only when fused with cellular metabolism; it is impossible to capture them in their dormant or inactive state, a stage which Duff aptly refers to as "undead." In their undead state, viruses are virtual as they exist liminally only in terms of their potential activity; at the same time, they exist as objects when they are immortalized by means of visual representation. Thus, viruses are both entities and events: technically, they are characterized by different material states transitioning when conditions are advantageous (i.e., the virion comes in contact with a compatible host). Yet, static imaging is the preferred way to display them.

For Duff, exploring the viral becomes a way to evoke all the forms through which viruses exist: as potentiality, as object, and as movement. Duff mentions how the process leading to the creation of the actual bruised piece of tissue (the artifact) is as important (if not more important) as the display of the artifact in the gallery. The virus is both an entity displayed in the gallery and an event (or even a series of events). Duff is especially interested in making sure that the process leading to the artifact is evident. Her meticulous work of documentation is an attempt to open the gallery to the activity of the lab, a space where important things happen, but suddenly disappear when it is time to show the "results" in public.

Reproducing, or at least giving a sense of the dynamic and ephemeral, multiplicitous, and relational nature of the virus is an operation that requires—at least partially—the rejection of some main tenets of representationalism. This can be done through Barad's "agential realism," by paying particular attention to the "energetic side of matter" (Hui 2015), or to the fact that there is no individual matter, but many matters, which are dynamically and mutually constituting (Barad 2014).

Using the principles of tissue culture engineering, Duff transplanted viral host cells onto skin in vitro. The inscription of the virus into the skin was made visible thanks to "immunohistochemical staining," a process that reveals a reaction of antibodies in the skin cells through color dyes. With this procedure, the virus manifests visually, becoming present in the form of bruises in transition and expansion across the skin. Duff observes that the virus exists as an invisible viral entity throughout the study of tissue culture, the purchase of the virus, and its preparation. The final product, the bruised skin, is an objectified inscription of the virus, and not a manifestation of the entire process preceding the moment of revelation to the public. Yet, the constant transformation of the virus appearing and disappearing across the tissue is the vivid proof of the intra-action, or the entangled state (or states) of the virus inside its host.

It is important to note that Duff and Berrigan, with their work, do not mean to "produce or prove a theory or hypothesis, let alone to create a canon of artifacts and documentation" (Duff 2009, 42). In other words, their work is not meant either to compete or to substitute the work of the scientist. In their comprehensive exploration of what viruses do and how they behave, Duff and Berrigan's works do expose the difficulties of representing the full significance and functions of viruses in one single image or one individual object. By creating different installations and by revealing viruses through different media and formats, they also show the range and diversity of instruments and techniques—as well as the "behind the scenes"—employed by scientists and professionals to visualize viruses. In both Duff's and Berrigan's works, viruses take multiple forms and span across a temporal range that documents all the processes needed to prepare, examine, and visualize them.

Duff and Berrigan did not invent new methods of scientific visualization. Instead, they embraced and incorporated existing visualization conventions into their artistic practices. In order to create these works, the two artists learnt the language of biology. Their presence and legitimacy as artists researching in a lab or in a medical context come from a solid knowledge and an at least partial acceptance of the rules governing scientific protocols and research procedures.

By accepting the operations and conventions of science, Duff and Berrigan were active participants in the biopolitical paradigm that subjects bìos to politics in attempting to tame and reproduce the virus, the object to the scientific instrument; the tendency to exercise control over a seemingly aleatory body. In fact, their work is evidence of the persistence of the models, assumptions, and tropes utilized by science and commonly understood at a more general level. The use of these models is, however, necessary if the desire is to communicate with a crowd that may be equally accustomed or unfamiliar with science.

The main issue here is not whether Duff and Berrigan's works can be considered legitimate or scientifically sound examples of visualization (though their protocols and mastery of instruments is) but how elements in their work can add to or help illuminate visualization more critically. In the end, by simultaneously embracing and adding to the current practice of visualization, and by undoing its consistency, they trigger reflection about its value and uses.

I believe that the significance of these two works can be better appreciated when we analyze how the technical and the aesthetic seamlessly intersect in the visualization of viruses. By zooming in onto the virus as if it was the only item in a Petri dish (a tendency I call the in vitro approach in Chapter 4), science illustrators create 3D models that combine different research data and modulate different aesthetic principles to build "an identity for the virus," in order to grab the public's attention. The goal is to communicate scientific information as well as to make viewers pay more attention to the virus. As Eckert states when asked whether the image she and Higgins created for the CDC has become the identity of the outbreak: "I keep saying people needed a face for the virus. They needed a way to make something complex tangible and I think it did" (Berlin 2020).

Seeing as Knowledge and the Technico-Aesthetic Image

For Jean Trumbo "There is a variety of potential uses for visual representation as a learning tool[.] The scientist, the science communicator, and the public use visual images in many of these capacities, as news and information about science is made available" (Trumbo 2000). Most visual representations of viruses sit at the convergence and are manifestations of social and cultural understandings of the objects represented that are based on a specific history of seeing and visual representation. Different circumstances and diverse publics can result in a great variety of visual outputs. Never has this practice made itself so clear like during the COVID-19 pandemic.

The operation of running raw data and blurry images through processing software and turning them into usable and meaningful pictures, Pauwels suggests, qualifies these products of visualization as "artifact" or as "creative works" (Pauwels 2006). Illustrators master software and combine different research findings to achieve visual renderings that not only provide sound information about a virus but also make these renderings memorable and even iconic. Technical details and aesthetics merge in the practice of visualization. For instance, the illustration created by Eckert and Higgins (Figure 9) posted as a public domain image on the CDC website reveals SARS-CoV-2 in sharp "red on grey color scheme, with orange and yellow accents." A "beauty spot," as media artist Stephanie Rothenberg observes in her video essay (The Beauty Spot 2020). "Does it all come down to this? this spiky blob that has been burned into the retina of all of us?" Rothenberg asks, referring to the iconic and now ubiquitous imagery of the coronavirus that, no matter what color scheme or technique it sports, has made its way across different audiences and different professional realms. In her playful video, she explains how although the "spiky blob" representing the coronavirus always remains the same, the color schemes and the slight shape variations are always different following various styles adapted to situations, audience, and message. Styles may remind us of familiar objects: a "kids' toy," a "psychedelic acne commercial," a "bad eighties aesthetics or an architecture parametric design thing etc ... " (Rothenberg 2020).

But style is not solely responsible for model variations. "Building a 3-D model of a complete virus like SARS-CoV-2 in molecular detail requires a mix of research, hypothesis and artistic license" (Falconieri Hays 2020), proclaims Falconieri in an essay where she explains how she created her version of the coronavirus 3D model (Figure 10). The resulting illustration is admittedly an in-progress model, as at the time—summer 2020—she had to "make best-guess decisions based on the evidence available," including selecting and combining different research by different labs and incorporating data and imagery from previous coronavirus when such information was still not available for SARS-CoV-2. In a series created for the *New York Times*, commented on by science journalist Carl Zimmer, cinematic techniques and state-of-the-art graphics are employed to turn simulations into innovative interactives that capture viewers' attention and please their aesthetics sensibilities. In this case, the journalist worked with web developers, who delivered a series of one-page interactive articles where the virus is prominently displayed, giving the impression of mobility and dynamicism (Corum et al. 2020; Corum and Zimmer 2020; Zimmer 2020).

Cinematic display, bright colors meticulously chosen for attention, aesthetic licenses. Clive Cazeaux argues that the scientific image is a construction, consisting of a series of mutually defining "intra-actions," in which "the object depicted cannot be separated from the technologies depicting it" (Cazeaux 2015). This situation, adds Natasha Myers, calls attention to the "impossibility of disentangling experimenters from the objects, apparatuses, and practices they engage to draw phenomena into view" (Myers 2015, 130).

The visualization of the unseen constitutes one of the foundations of today's notion of knowledge. José van Dijck (van Dijck 2005) has observed how visualization instruments are closely related to media technologies on different levels: their technological developments often go hand in hand, as the emergence of visualization instruments has followed technological innovation and ubiquitous digitization; media increasingly function as intermediaries for knowledge and, specifically, medical visualization knowledge. In addition, media and visualization converge in the production of visual spectacle.

The establishment of this relation finds its roots in the belief that seeing is a key to knowledge. The seventeenth and eighteenth centuries produced myriads of visual metaphors, including the ones that emphasized the role of light in the acquisition of better vision, something necessary in order to put an end to (intellectual) blindness. While these metaphors mostly referred to intellectual enhancement, exhorting the educated individual and the scientist to instruct the confused and "intellectually impaired" masses, they were no doubt inspired by the technical breakthroughs in optics and by a recovered confidence in the role of observation in the natural sciences. Visual representations do rationalize the object. "The scientific notions of 'objectivity'" (van Loon 2002a, 112), van Loon observes, ".. have always (or at least since Plato) been ordained by the principle of visibility." If, ".. in order to be credible, the object must be observable .." (109), then, new methods and technologies of visibility come to assist in assigning a visual form to viruses. Visualization isolates something immaterial or difficult to grasp, it extracts its crucial information, it processes such information, and turns it into a—tangible—object.

The abilities of new optic instruments (the telescope and the microscope) to produce visual evidence not only facilitated new discoveries but were also crucial in demonstrating theories and mathematical hypotheses in natural philosophy and astronomy that had emerged during the scientific revolution. Observation had taken on a new role in demonstrating and adjusting the Copernican-inspired heliocentric model of the universe, whose main principles were based on mathematics. Galileo's major discoveries were possible thanks to the telescope (whose main function as a trade and military instrument he had adapted for his astronomic observations). The microscope, which enthusiasts such as Robert Hooke (Hooke 1780) swore "brought about an improvement of the organ of sight" (especially in the wake of Antonie van Leeuwenhoek's dissemination of the portable "simple microscope"), produced similar developments. For most of these early adopters, optical instruments multiplied the resources available for observation, allowing for more and more complex discoveries (Schickore 2009).

The art of making one's discoveries visible to others had been a key feature of scientific research even before Copernicus. However, as Bernard Le Bovier de Fontenelle reminds us: "All philosophy is based on two things only: curiosity and poor eyesight … The trouble is, we want to know more than what we can see" (de Fontenelle 2000). The encounter between the need to "see better" described by de Fontenelle and the "art of making visible" was complicated by an increased popularization of science. The Enlightenment, Stafford points out, was "extremely sensitive to the multiple ways in which one's impression of reality might become corrupted" (Stafford 1996, 9). As discoveries are disseminated and instruments become available to a wider population, there appears also a proliferation of misleading information, quack science, plagiarism, and importantly, varieties of visual representations and aesthetic manipulations of the images produced. Nevertheless, for those in the Enlightenment era, the newer instruments that were becoming available to a larger amount of people, from natural scientists to private enthusiasts, were increasingly trusted as being able to provide more accurate and precise evidence than it was possible to gain with the naked eye.

With the gradual introduction of scientific instruments that partially mechanized the process of seeing, by visually reproducing, recording and increasing amounts of information, came an acceptance that mechanical visual aids were the ultimate solution for the problem of subjective judgment (Daston and Galison 1992, 81). This way of thinking derives from an increasing trust in quantity and quantification, two connected but distinct qualities that have dominated many scientific disciplines since the seventeenth century: First, there is a belief that the larger the amount of data collected and aggregated from a given phenomenon, the more accurate the conclusions will be. This confirms the widely held idea that visualization is simply a "transformer directing a deluge of data" rather than "a form of data in itself" (Turnbull 2015, 73). Second, the quantifications available from scientific research have been seen as offering better, more specific details about phenomena that can be provided by other disciplines, such as poetry and the other arts, which are not providing quantifiable data (Dror 2001).

Historically, "the division between a sensuous, pleasurable, or merely curious watching and a rational, tasking, language-driven observation arose during the eighteenth century" (Stafford 1996, 2). An entertaining scientific image of a microscopic organism ("enjoyable watching") could potentially distract the viewer from the specific information ("exacting observation") provided by the image. However, entertaining features drew attention to the image and were typical practice in eighteenth-century scientific illustrations, since the objects depicted were seen as the "spectacle of nature," and as the work of God (Hooke 1780). The scientist's approach to depicting objects seen through the microscope appeared to be more like that of a voyeur than a detached viewer. In that sense, the practice of observing organisms through a lens was not unlike the activity of peering through a hole at something forbidden. The activity married, in a sense, a prurient attitude toward the dirty and base, yet marvelous and fantastic organisms under scrutiny with rigorous scientific observation of the invisible unknown where "mysterious animalcules with unexpected powers could be not only watched under the enlarging lens, but controlled and directed, even as they rushed by" (Stafford 1993a, 110).

Today, microscopy and scientific visualization are fully embedded in a system that mixes and exploits, on the one hand, technical information and "entertainment," and on the other hand, well-established visual tropes and innovations that move away from these tropes. The more scientists incorporate new technologies of representation and media display into their research, the better able they are to record natural phenomena, which results in them being more easily able to move their findings "from the laboratory to the auditorium," producing a so-defined "cinema of scientific vernacularization" (Landecker 2006). This ability improves the dissemination of images and information to a much wider audience, including both fellow scientists, who are competing for attention, visibility, and eventually more funding, and the general public, who are more likely to be attracted to imagery that is easy to grasp and is appealing (or frightening) to the eye.

Unsurprisingly, these technologies, techniques, and effects are increasingly shared by members of the art and entertainment industries, who use these methods and technologies in their artistic, cinematic, and narrative works. Whereas science borrows cinema's techniques in order to secure interest from a variety of individuals, the film industry appropriates sequences and data from the sciences in order to assume a kind of legitimacy and to give the impression of realism or veracity. As a result, it is not uncommon to see some of the popular constructs that characterize our perception of a scientific phenomenon being equally developed as a collaboration between the film industry and the scientific community (Milburn 2002). Scientific and statistical information about infectious diseases becomes mixed in Hollywood movies, while scientific films and other visual expressions use cinematic techniques to illustrate and disseminate specific findings.

The recent interactive pieces written by Zimmer and published on the *New York Times* website meant for online consumption are an excellent example of the way cinematic techniques are used to achieve a number of goals: to provide information about the pandemic and the virus causing it; to attract a larger readership with a skillfully designed, interactive page; to evoke reactions of awe and marvel at the speed of scientific research in a time of crisis and at the graphic gimmicks accompanying it. Similarly, Eckart and Higgins were tasked to create a model that would provide a ".. detailed, realistic-looking 3D sphere that conveys immediacy and clarity." At the same time, the model had to be "uniquely CDC in appearance, but easily reproducible." In other words, when it came to colorizing the model, they couldn't use any color schemes, but instead had to adapt their design to the branding colors chosen by the CDC to disseminate their literature about the virus. This move ascertained that the model was easily associated with a reputable and official source and would assure consistency. Using Cinema 4D, Falconieri had to make the decision to add a stem to the coronavirus protein. In recent research on SARS-CoV-2 "scientists know that these regions exist, and what amino acids (protein building blocks) they include, but have not yet been able to observe their arrangement in 3-D space" (Falconieri Hays 2020). She eventually chose to follow the direction of the team at the Amaro lab to include such detail, making her model a bit different from other existing models, a choice that has both a scientific and aesthetic rationale, and is part of her model signature as a scientific illustrator. Once again, the resulting model contained scientific information unavoidably packaged in aesthetic. But dismissing this effort (as well as the efforts made by Eckart and Higgings at CDC and Falconieri at *Scientific American*) as mere spectacle would miss the significance of a (visualization and publishing) practice that has to rely on both technological innovation and aesthetic strategies in order to receive the attention and the visibility it deserves, as well as to stand out and defend itself from unauthorized or unreliable sources.

If technical images only reproduce selected information about the virus, then the various arbitrary forms produced are signs of the application of curatorial and aesthetic choices. Partially drawing from the awareness of this distinction, the discourse disparaging certain images as "misleading illusions without the guidance of discourse" (Stafford 1993a, 2) still holds true. Despite the increasingly important role played by images in science since the eighteenth century, their significance as independent sources of knowledge is still treated with suspicion. Yet, images have become a must-have item in scientific research; they attract and fascinate the general public; they help the scientist and the science team/lab obtain the visibility they need to attract funding; and they symbolize a gesture of openness toward the public.

Control and Transformation

Scientific visualization is typified by incessant innovation. However, researchers appear to be unable to reach a definite agreement about how viruses should be represented. Looking at the process of visualization and the way in which the images found in science journals and popular science magazines are produced offers clues about the scientific management of viruses. It also reveals how the figurations of viruses that consumers, in both the scientific community and amongst the general public, are invited to accept, are, in turn, shaped by the cultural tropes and collective narratives already in place. These established views necessarily affect how viruses are displayed.

While the contemporary goal-oriented practice of microscopy has maintained an approach to the microscopic as a territory that can be colonized and dissected, objectified and manipulated, the coexistence of the "aesthetic" and the "instrumental," the "entertaining" and the "educational" confirms that the attempts (of politics) to govern the vital (bìos) described earlier by Esposito will never be accomplished. This is not to say that science has not been successful in achieving accurate or precise visualization. It means that given the qualities of viruses and given the prevalent epistemological principles that characterize this practice, visualization will always produce images that are technologically sophisticated and precisely drafted, but also partial, not because they are missing something, but because they must make the decision to leave something behind.

Although researchers may share the scientific urge to constrain, regulate, and control visual expressions, individually they possess different agendas (different public, branding, the need to sell a subscription, the need to achieve scholarly visibility, etc.), and so a variety of approaches to visualization are necessary to sustain specific research questions and to adapt the imagery to different publics and situations. To communicate such agendas, these visual expressions are compelled, to some degree, to conform to established aesthetics. By the same token, the acceptance of the conventional is constantly undermined by a desire and a need to find new ways of display. As a result, frequent introductions of innovative elements (technological and conceptual) can and do occur.

Contesting the rules regarding the representation of the microscopic, whether it involves scientists, artist, or others, is evidence that visualization is heavily mediated by, and not severed from, our cultural assumptions and notions of seeing. The apparent tension between the attempt to regulate visualization and the constant emergence of variations is not produced by a failure to separate the purely technical from the aesthetic, but by a necessity to accommodate different intertwined positions, including technical innovation and cultural assumptions, the very material qualities of the viruses and the way scientific instruments and technologies manipulate them.

Berrigan and Duff are not above this contest. Their practices reveal an awareness that providing alternative forms of representation involves acknowledging the general trends that dominate scientific visualization. To put it in Stengers's words, they had to act as innovators to "transform conditions into constraints, in other words, not to submit to existing relations of force but to rework the implications, at least partially" (Stengers 2010, 43). This is made obvious by their direct engagement with the practice of science and with the existing models that characterize the visualization of viruses. Breaking these rules does not, however, involve a simple abrupt disruption of the status quo; rather, it includes, also, a relocating of visualizations outside the lab and an assembling of them differently. Completely ignoring the models of visualization that exist would be a mistake and would detach the works of the artists from the practice of science; the absence of direct references to known practices would result in the loss of their message (Rasmussen 1999).

Berrigan and Duff use the same models (derived from databases) employed in traditional scientific research. Berrigan's reproductions of the structure of the hepatitis C virus, the chocolate candies, and the geodesic shelter, derive from models found on the PDB. Her use of two forms to represent the virus helps to underline the fact that it is, in fact, an unstable entity; likewise, her letters to the hepatitis C virus render it both ephemeral and vivid.

Duff uses tissue culture protocols to produce her viral tattoos. In performing this work, she realized that although the presence of the virus can only be viewed when it is made visible in the form of a bruise, it has, nonetheless, been present as an invisible and virtual entity since the beginning of her relationship with it. Documentation of the early stages of the viral infection is necessary, therefore, to provide a complete picture of the artist's realization. And so, the documentation and the image of the effect of the virus on the skin are complementary. The first is not secondary to the second, as the virus manifests through both practices: "Each practice is mutually reliant on the other to evoke a complex threshold of live encounters" (Duff 2009, 38). In fact, "the interrelation between performance and documentation can be seen as viral" itself (39).

Importantly, the two artists did not erase already existing practices and protocols but added to them. This, they achieve by combining multiple components in their work—the installation collecting chocolates and the geodesic domes, in combination with informative material about hepatitis C in Berrigan's work, information about the process leading to the final appearance of the viruses in Duff's, work along with the tattooed skin as well, by merging performance and archival/informative items (the process of culturing and transposing the lentivirus in Duff's work), by presenting traditional material using unusual media (as in Berrigan's chocolate instead of plastic, or plaster). In doing so, they show how any given model, if taken individually, while useful to pinpoint specific aspects of them, is unable to convey the multiple articulations of viruses. However, each model becomes a source of inspiration, a point of departure and an invitation to explore further.

Their works epitomize the combination of the "aesthetic" and the "instrumental," the "entertaining" and the "educational." They include explanatory pamphlets and documentary narratives, showing, once again, that images can't by themselves serve as explanatory tools. Visitors viewing their works do not find a single picture, or a virus floating in a void; instead, they are presented with a multiplicity of things: objects and equally legitimate and scientifically sound documents that testify to the nature of viruses as multiplicitous and embedded.

In addition to highlighting the difficulties that scientists and laboratory technicians experience in visualizing viruses, the complex works of Duff and Berrigan reveal how traditional modes of visualization can be reconfigured to provide fresh perspectives.

The location of these artists at the crossroads of the sciences and the arts puts them in a privileged position, giving them the freedom to reveal with greater clarity those problematic assumptions that characterize the study and representation of the invisible. Thus, while not directly revolutionizing or proposing new ways of seeing, these works do initiate (for those who want to learn) a process of transformation in how we understand and approach "objects" as volatile and elusive as viruses.

4

From a Distance

In the previous chapter, I examined the complex process of visualization from the preparation of the virus specimen to graphic representation and publication. During this process, the obligation to showcase the virus as one image vis-à-vis its material dynamicity, the difficulty in reconciling the need to respect scientific conventions and the pressures to pursue technological innovation, and the technical and aesthetic negotiations leading to visualization contribute to the variety and heterogeneity of this practice. In this chapter, I explore another function of imaging: the technologies and techniques used to examine and process viruses create a physical and perceived distance between the viewer and the object analyzed. This distance is in part produced by practical needs. For example, as the viral object is represented with increasing minutia, it undergoes a process of geometrification, resembling less a natural organism and more a computer-generated being. In addition, distance between the object and the observer is created to simultaneously control and protect (or protect the observer from) the object. In the case of computer viruses, visualizations and illustrations are forms of interpellation, as they identify, isolate, and zero in on an entity that is anything but tangible.

Going back to the way an image is presented publicly, there is growing awareness that the scientific illustrations of viral molecules produced today are comprised of several technological layers, and diverse research—an awareness that, according to Ornes, has been reinforced by the coronavirus pandemic, thanks to the well-researched models of the virus published by the CDC, *Scientific American*, and other well-publicized sources (Ornes 2021). However, there is still a lingering tendency to interpret technologies of visualization through an epistemological paradigm already established in the late eighteenth century, as "transparent, neutral intermediaries between the scientist and nature" (Pasveer 2006, 43). Take well-known viruses like coronavirus, HIV, Ebola, with their distinctive characteristics and their diminutive size that makes them invisible: the illustrations that we see in the news or in science publications both are and are not the virus. They have been edited, reconstructed, and enhanced, yet, they are the only illustrations we have. Here, two mechanisms contribute in rendering the technologies filtering these viruses transparent: first, the mechanical objectivity produced by the instrument substitutes "the machine for the human sensory apparatus" (Daston and Galison 2010, 43). As Myers observes, rendering molecules as machines not only enables practitioners to visualize and intervene in molecular worlds, but it also turns the rendering into a machine itself. The transformation occurs through a process of materialized refiguration where the metaphor (of the molecular rendering being equated to a machine) and the material formation of the molecular content of the virus collapse during the very performative act of rendering (Myers 2014).

In this chapter, I also turn my attention to how seeing as knowing fulfills a cultural need for taming and protecting oneself from the unknown: although technologies are often perceived as transparent, they still separate the object observed from the observer, serving a fundamental protective role. Seeing becomes knowing through a lens, a screen, a page on a magazine, without touching. With the unknown being associated historically with fear, darkness and not being able to see as, itself, a generator of fear, seeing becomes exorcism against darkness; technologies as tools to prepare, filter, manipulate, and present viruses create a safe distance between the observer and the object and act as a protection against the unknown and against the threat caused by the virus.

In this chapter, computer viruses make a comeback. While computer virus visualizations are notably less crucial to the understanding of malware, they currently manifest interesting new strategies of display that, on the one hand, connect them to the networks and the social and technical environment surrounding them; on the other hand, they help better elucidate the notion of distancing as control, defense, and protection.

In this chapter, I will continue to focus on transdisciplinary artists Tagny Duff and Caitlin Berrigan and will introduce two recent works by Laura Splan. In three different ways, the artists connect "hidden artifacts of biotechnology to everyday domains" (Splan 2021). As explored in Chapter 3, Duff's *Living Viral Tattoos* make the lentivirus visible thanks to a process of staining and infection. Importantly, through a combination of performance (the durational performance of the virus walking across the tissue) and documentation of the processes that must be utilized in order to render viruses visible, her work also makes technologies visible. Berrigan's reproduction of the virus in different forms, as lace capsid-dome, as delicious, yet insidious, chocolate treat, as a series of statistics, draws a map of its different faces according to how it affects individuals or manifests itself.

Splan's 2004 *Doilies* (SARS) and her recent animations of the protein spikes of SARS-CoV-2 reveal the mediated nature of biomolecular visualization as well as its protective function by reproducing the virus using the familiar craft of lace and by turning the visualization software used to give the virus a visible form into a medium to manipulate the proteins of the virus aesthetically. The virus becomes both a familiarized object and a tame body, which can be virtually manipulated and shaped at will. Manipulation and rendition using software or craft don't change the nature of the virus. Doilies are familiar objects often hiding insidious (domestic) violence. The virus remains a shapeshifting trickster figure (Akomolafe et al. 2020) not to be trusted.

Viruses and the Unknown

"Who knows everything, fears nothing" (Virilio 2000, 54): By quoting Goebbels, Paul Virilio indicated how knowledge, at least in the West, is perceived as the ultimate form of control, which he saw as a continuation and realization of the myth of the frontier. In fact, achieving knowledge/control can be interpreted as a race or a quest for expansion beyond the frontiers of the humanly visible or beyond the defined territory of the physical. Virilio assigns quite an aggressive connotation to knowledge, not only because it references the infamous Reich Minister of Propaganda of Nazi Germany, but also because it gestures to the project of civilization, conquest, and colonization of the so-called "founding fathers." Merritt Roe Smith, in the 1994 classic essay on technological determinism, famously illustrated how knowledge is both connected with progress and the development of new technologies, and how this notion of progress is inseparable from aggressive expansion. The 1870 painting *American Progress* by Michael Gast is a vivid testimony to this particular belief: in it, progress, portrayed as a woman, advances inexorably, pushing her body ahead, further West, into unknown territories, bringing with her communication and transportation technologies as the signs of civilization, and destroying everything she finds in her way, including other forms of knowledge (Smith 1994). Knowledge, per se, does not acquire relevance unless it is channeled through the conventional tools, the methodologies and procedures, and the language that will validate it. If we follow these principles, to successfully explore viruses means to remove the boundaries that delimit the frontier of the unknown.

The unknown, explains Virilio, is a continuously shifting horizon to be conquered and turned into the known. To do this, risky explorations have been undertaken to push the unknown further away, and increasingly sophisticated technological instruments (the microscope and the telescope) have been fabricated to conquer the infinitely small and the extremely far away. Exploring and observing with success the protein configuration of viruses, or, in information technologies, being able to detect and break down the basic code that constitutes computer viruses and worms should equally lead to the achievement of a certain degree of control over them. Only then, and, importantly, only by following appropriate technical and discipline-specific rules, can viruses be fully known and mastered. It is implied that using better tools to “see” viruses (i.e., by extracting more accurate data out of increasingly mechanized and quantified processes) would ultimately liberate us from viral fear.

A fitting example proving Virilio’s point is the 2017 Nobel prize in chemistry, which was awarded to three scientists for “their pioneering work developing new methods of visualizing biomolecules such as those in the Zika virus” (Krämer 2017; Vonberg 2017). The three scientists were praised for having developed and perfected a cryo-electron microscope able to “decipher almost any biomolecule’s structure” and a “conquest” that required “determination” (Krämer 2017) as well as a good dose of funding and technological equipment.

With his notion of knowing as moving the horizon that separates the known from the unknown, Virilio confirms the centrality of sight as the major sense we rely on to put a face to the unknown and the undefined. Card, Mckinlay, and Schneiderman (1999), in an early text introducing data visualization, clearly connect knowing to seeing: “We try to make our ideas ‘clear’, to bring them into ‘focus’ to ‘arrange’ our thoughts. The ubiquity of visual metaphors in describing cognitive processes hints at a nexus of relationship between what we see and what we think” (1).

Metaphors evoking the notion of knowing as conquering the unknown are used equally in the biological sciences and in computer sciences. In both cases, viruses must be known (often visually, where sometimes the word “see” is used metaphorically) before they can be domesticated. Companies and research units involved in the field of visualization describe their activities as being “the final frontier” (Coy 1996; IN-VSEE 2008). Searching the shifting horizon means constantly striving for something that moves farther and farther away. In computing, understanding viruses literally equals putting up a defense against them. To single out and to erect limits means also to minimize their impact and damaging potential.

While seeing might allow for the uncovering and understanding of the unknown, the inability to see is disorienting. “*Peur toujours, peur partout*”(Bauman 2006, 2): with these words, Sygmunt Bauman brings back Febvre’s description of “the experience of living in XVI century Europe,” when fear was evoked by darkness, “which started just on the other side of the hut door and wrapped the world beyond the farm fence … ” (2). Darkness does not necessarily harbor any threat. However, it is the natural locus of uncertainty and mystery, the place where anything can happen (4). The convention of portraying viruses as if they were emerging from a dark void somehow evokes this uncertainty.

By turning viruses into images, visual representation challenges the domain of the unknown. At the same time, instruments and chemical processes assist and mediate visual representation, building a protection against the obscure domain of the unknown. Scientific instruments, Turner observes, “are, after all, ideas made brass” (Turner 1972, 1). Pictures, maps, and models constitute different ways of making the invisible visible, the abstract into the tangible to bring order to the indeterminacy of chaos and to "neutralize and contain what provoked anxiety and distress" (Bauman 2006).

In a sense, there is an affinity between modern utopias and the new frontier: "insofar as real spaces elsewhere have been exhausted, it is necessary to find new kinds of place and frontier that sustain the needs of the modern imaginary" (15). With its current richness, the industry involved in assigning a visual appearance to viruses embraces this notion of knowledge. While visualizing or illustrating a virus satisfies the curiosity of imagining and materializing the unknown, it also encapsulates the anxiety that the object visualized generates (Robins 1996, 58). The act of seeing, and the technologies built to see serve both the functions of imagining and re-presenting, as well as the act of erecting a defense against the demon of the unknown.

Robins explains how technology constitutes an obvious, and therefore often unnoticeable, component in the formation of visuals. It is called upon as a protection that transcends and potentially exorcises the fearful chaos of the world. Technology brings in focus, enhances performance, and amplifies vision, all by filtering and ordering the world through digital code, interface, lenses, receptacles, etc. It is supposedly able to make every object visible, yet maintaining it substantially virtual and, importantly, keeping it at a safe distance.

Instruments involved in microscopy, digital technologies such as 3D rendering and molecular visualization software, as well as the negotiating agency of the many individuals involved in this endeavor equally contribute to the study, ordering, and visual representation of the virus. The apparatuses, the screens, the data encoding contributing to making viruses intelligible stand between the viewer and the now made-visible, yet physically separate, entity. Technologically mediated visions prevent us from being in direct contact with, to purposely touch, its reality (Robins and Webster 1999).

Interestingly, for Robins and Webster, this approach is not much different from the functions of today's ubiquitous surveillance cameras. Surveillance cameras see from a safe distance without being seen. It is not much different from the tendency of Modernist architecture to use glass walls as it "sought to erase what we may call the city of touch, and in its place to construct the glass city" (19). Its fundamental objective is the creation "of transparency," aspiring to the idea of universal panopticism, through which it seems possible to "achieve order, and consequently master, the urban space" (20). Both the technologies used and the very methods employed in the process of visualization support a notion of knowledge that privileges this act of "seeing from a safe distance." Like the glass window separating the observer from the observed, the appearance of viruses is never experienced directly, but through a number of sometimes barely unnoticeable filters.

The situation is no different when the virus contemplated is a computer virus, made up of nothing but code. Users barely (or never) become aware of this code; it is hidden and it is of no use to them in order to use a computer with proficiency. In place of struggling with code, users install antivirus software to protect themselves from sudden malware attacks. These sophisticated programs make unnecessary any attempts by users to seek DIY solutions that could potentially endanger not only their personal computer but an entire network. These "easy to use" virus protection programs isolate and hide suspicious code bundles that may cause problems away from the user, by placing them in quarantine. These programs run in the background, becoming visible only during upgrades. They offer users an interface that seems transparent, but, in fact, leaves its inner structure opaque. In protecting users from external dangers and from themselves, virus protection programs distance users from the realities affecting them while at the same time concealing their own complexity (Van Den Eede 2011).

The In Vitro Approach and Computer Malware

Technologies appear to separate objects from the viewer, creating images that are only partially tied to those objects' supposedly physical form. By subjecting—the abstract or invisible—entity to a series of mechanical and chemical processes, by combining information from different sources to form a whole as it is done with the molecular models of the coronavirus, and by creating models of computer viruses that assign a visual appearance to abstract code based on familiar images and forms, we are translating, hence re-creating and transforming viruses. What we call the object is an entity that is always already transformed, the result of a "mutual constitution of entangled agencies" (Barad 2014).

As observed on other occasions, the entanglement of viruses with the external world is often dismissed, because it is distractive, and when it is present, it is viewed as being the product of pure mechanics (Bennett 2010). The virus is portrayed as part of a static environment. This approach reflects an approach typical of lab science after Pasteur. The scientist separates the entity studied from its milieu and moves it to a controlled environment, such as a Petri dish where its growth can be optimally analyzed. The same "in vitro approach" can be observed when a forensic analysis is called to reconstruct and simulate the behavior of computer viruses. In such cases, the condition of the host is observed and simulated in relation to malware before and after the digital infection. In microbiology, many operations reinforce this modus operandi: the variety of procedures such as fixation, dehydration, infiltration, and embedding, the staining and coating described earlier, so that the microscope can fix it in its current state. While these processes facilitate the identification of the virus, they destroy the crucial qualities that make the virus a virus, that is, its dynamic nature and adaptive behavior, its connection and enmeshing with its host and the other entities that normally float around it.

The existence of computer viruses and malware as parasitic agents that become active only when they are launched inside an existing computer environment (the host computer), and when they are triggered by an external event (such as the opening of an attachment), is generally not visible. No visual representation of viruses shows their relationship with, and their dependence on, such an event. Illustrations created to show the merging of malware and host computer usually portray one single virus already inside the host, emulating the situation of the virus in a digital Petri dish ready to be scrutinized through a virtual microscope, but omit the process of infection that has allowed the virus to enter the host.

The in vitro approach in computing is exemplified by the concept of the honeypot, a computer or computer system ".. intended to mimic likely targets of cyberattacks" (*What Is a Honeypot?*, 2020). A honeypot is devoted to capturing and trapping malware. The scope is to detect attacks or deflect them from a legitimate target, or to gain information about how cybercriminals operate. This strategy isolates in order to study malware and in order to expedite the dissemination of new patches and solutions (Galloway and Thacker 2007, 107; Kaspersky n.d.). Once trapped inside this virtual environment, the computer virus can be analyzed and simulations (visual or not) of its transformation and spread can be generated. The main purpose of the honeypot is to create a safe environment for experimentation, analogous to the safe environment of the lab. Visual representations of the behavioral patterns of viruses are based on the above premises.

Visual representations of malware spread have become possible thanks to the introduction of new data visualization tools. These visuals often take the form of colorful maps. They are often animated, to simulate the extensiveness and the intensity of the spread. Most of these visualizations tend to display general or global trends, that is, malware spread across the world or across one or more networks. It is rare to find images or sequences documenting the process of intrusion and infection inside one single machine, and the ensuing triggering of the security software. One such example is an early simulation produced by F-Secure, a security company based in Finland. Drawn from the popular TV series *CSI (Crime Scene Investigation)* popular in the early 2000s, FS-CSI (F-Secure Crime Scene Investigation) was presented as a simulation via an animated sequence of how viruses infect data on one hard drive. According to the analysts presenting the simulation based on the analysis of forensic data, the animation "[r]ecords data before and after the [viral] sample is run and then compares the two for changes: the intermediate stage, that is, the process that has led to the infection is, then, guessed, based on the evidence provided by the previous two states" (F-Secure 2007). Its general goal was to easily intercept and visually underscore the areas mostly damaged: "Instead of looking at lines of code, we are looking at a graphical picture of what the malware has done to your system. This is something we have had to do in the lab to keep up with the challenge of all the malware we receive and improve the way we work" (F-Secure 2007), said Patrick Runald, a security specialist at F-Secure. Although the visual animation is technically not necessary for the simulation, it provides a more immediate clue of where the intrusion is located.

While this in vitro forensic procedure may lead to an increased understanding of the impact of the virus on the computer system and of the effectiveness of the security software against the virus, its focus tends to lie on the computer system itself. In fact, as the goal of the security industry is to protect and preserve computer systems, the study zooms into the affected machine and does not extend to the entire network.

Boundary Crossing and Boundary Building: Dancing between Authentic and Artificial

We know that the physical appearance usually attributed to viruses does not originate from direct observation but is the fruit of a convergence of different analyses, interpretations, and assumptions speculating about what viruses might look like. The technologies used in visualization confirm such evidence by capturing and selecting specific data that fit research questions and that can be seized thanks to existing research methods. In doing so, these technologies iterate the idea of knowledge as both boundary-crossing (to see better and beyond the existing limits, to pioneer new methods) and boundary-building (to protect and separate the object from the observer), thus reflecting and attempting to tame the anxieties and curiosity generated by viruses. Visual representational practices "[not only] represent a phenomenon that is observed in a historical and physical reality (thus implying iconical and indexical reality), but equally may include those ideographic activities that seek primarily to express ideas or relations and they have no material referent whatsoever (a combination of mimetic and expressive elements)" (Pauwels 2006, 6). When representing viruses, the existence of the referent (the virus constituted by RNA and proteins or a string of digital information) is only postulated. Thus, viruses are "enpresented," that is, their viral qualities (the virus as a virtual, transforming entity made of multiples, the event not yet occurred, but nonetheless existing) are made insightful, provisionally present (van Loon 2002a, 115).

The technological layers juxtaposed to retrieve information from and to obtain the image of a virus are not simply conceived to magnify and reproduce an object, but they are also technologies of display (116) geared toward running the "object-virus" through increasing rationalization. Simultaneously, they are technologies of disappearance, as they turn the unknown category of infectious agents into something somehow more "obscure," because it is only made visible thanks to the manipulation of media. Visualization and the rendering of scientific data then become a business of "producing scientific reality," rather than an operation to copy it (Lynch 2006, 40). According to Lynch, the production of scientific reality made by visualizations and 3D modeling fits the imperatives of science to make reality more understandable and accessible to a variety of individuals. It couldn't be otherwise, as reduction and simplification, coloring and refiguration are important keys toward facilitating the reading and the interpretation of the object. It may be the only way that technologies of seeing can realize their mission to create distance between viruses and the public, as well as to protect the observer by being able to give them a relative knowledge of the virus, while also giving the impression that any potential to-do damage is under control.

I would even go beyond this interpretation: by imagining the virus (and its representation) as "produced," we are still assuming that there must be, behind these artifacts, something (multiple, ephemeral, etc.) naturally existing. Yet, scientific visualization, illustrations, and other imagery pointing to the virus are all we can grasp: the virus comes to us always already mediated through technologies. The virus lies at the intersection of what we consider natural and what we deem artificial. As a matter of fact, the two aspects are not separable.

In addition to being the product of manipulation (aesthetic, functional, etc.), the operation of making viruses visible involves enpresentation as a necessity. The lengthy processes required to obtain an image testifies to this necessity. While the relatively recent development of instruments able to capture the energetic signals of viruses has given them a certain visibility, the operations required today to visualize their molecular content (preparation of specimens, visualization through the microscope and software manipulation) are still labor-intensive.

Going back to artistic interpretation of viruses, in *Living Viral Tattoos,* Duff explores the process of enpresentation described by Van Loon. In her work, technologies are made evident thanks to the integration of performance and documentation that records in detail the processes that must be utilized to render viruses visible. As I mentioned in the previous chapter, Duff had chosen to reveal the virus by inoculating a portion of pig and human tissue with lentivirus particles that would become visible in the form of bruises. The observer is able to identify the virus through its motion from cell to cell, while leaving a visible trace across the tissue and making the presence of the virus visible every time in a provisional form. Duff defines this provisional impression realized by technologies of seeing and chemical processes as an instance of the "viral." Her work, she notes, exposes "the act of encountering the viral, whether through the lens of laboratory science, medical science, or art" as an operation that "actualizes the threshold of liveliness between the virtual and its actualization through inscription" (Duff 2009, 40). In fact, viruses manifest through the mutual interrelation between performance and documentation, "each evoking the liveness of the other" (ibid.).

There is an interrelation between the culminating visual product and the processes required to obtain it; between the ephemeral and always changing appearance of the virus, and the meticulous operations devised to "tame" and "fixate" its elusive manifestations. With these operations unfolding and being documented throughout Duff's piece, the final stage leading to the appearance of the virus on human tissue is revealed as an incomplete action, as the bruises surfacing become mere marks of the ephemeral passage of the viral, as opposed to the viral as a pointer for the discrete entity.

While evoking similar awareness regarding the incompleteness of the models and other methods through which the hepatitis C virus is made present visually or otherwise, Berrigan's work goes in a different direction. In her multipart installation, the virus progressively extends its manifestations in space and in time, presenting itself through different forms, utilizing different media and materials, first as an enticing chocolate treat in the form of a molecular model, then as a welcoming geodesic dome, finally as a set of educational notes and a love letter evoking the complicated coexistence of the artist and the virus (Berrigan 2012). Rather than showing how the virus reproduces, during its manifestation, and the encounter between the virtual event and its actualization, Berrigan's work projects an idea of the virus as pervasive and profoundly connected to the individuals it affects (the observers, the artist, and individuals affected by the disease) by the material it wears each time and through which it is displayed (chocolate, fabric and laces, paper, etc.). The virus never takes an ultimate form but takes different forms according to how it affects individuals or manifests itself.

Inspired by the processes through which biotechnology makes microscopic agents such as viruses visible through molecular models and other schematics, Laura Splan's artworks offer new ways to make sense of scientific forms of representation by remaking them as everyday domestic artifacts, such as in the case of her 2004 *Doilies (SARS)*, which reproduces the molecular model of SARS as a common doily. In her recent 2020–21 work, *Unraveling*, she turned to the molecular visualization system PyMOL, a tool adopted by the Protein Data Bank to create and manipulate protein models. Splan started playing with the software during a residency at Integral Molecular – a biotechnology company developing innovative technologies and focusing on antibodies studies – becoming fascinated with its naming conventions and the modularity through which it operates. The function named "sculpting" in particular caught her attention as it evokes a sense of artistry, and it suggests that some form of sculptural manipulation is possible in the production of a model (Frattini 2021). During the interaction with this function, she would playfully and meticulously unravel (or unfold) the SARS-CoV-2 spike protein, engaging in interaction not only with the software interface, its functions, and its limitations, but also with the protein itself, creating "mesmerising pictorial and moving orchestrations of protein forms that determine biological function" (ibid.). Unlike scientists and technicians, she would use the software as if it was an experimental artistic tool, creating animations by recording her attempts to manipulate and reposition said spike proteins, just as a sculptor would do. The proteins would only move temporarily, or move in a "spastic way" immediately returning to their original position.

In both artworks—the doilies and the animations produced with PyMOL—Splan embraces the idea of mediatedness. With her doilies, she exposes the mechanism of mediation by translating software-produced molecular models into familiar objects. The regular and symmetric shape of the molecular model is easily reproduced using traditional lace. The fact that a familiar object such as the doily can reproduce a molecular model reveals how the virus exists and is made visible only as a mediated, manipulated object displaying symmetries and geometries that are much more complicated in nature.

The doily, Splan observes, is a decorative artifact associated with "familiarity and comfort of domesticity." At the same time, it is used to hide a scratch or stain on furniture. When it takes the form and appearance of a dangerous virus, it acts as a reminder of a—faraway and faint—real threat. The doily has a symbolic protective function both in its material role and in its reassuring appearance. Following the policies of "shelter in place" and the direct association of the domestic place to a literal safe place during the COVID-19 pandemic, the doily becomes a symbol of domesticity as protection (Splan 2021). In reality, as Anna Dumitriu's installation will demonstrate in the next chapter, the perceived protection provided by the domestic place hides insidious dangers: as people protect themselves from the virus by staying at home, they may become vulnerable to other threats, such as domestic violence or abusive relations. Span's doilies (Figure 15) hint at these hidden threats: these decorative items may be used to cover up stains and other flaws that cannot be seen unless they are removed or they are examined closely. In a way, a similar effect is produced when a virus is digitized and visualized using professional software: the resulting image is only meant to display a partial picture (Figure 16).

Splan's use of PyMOL to produce the *Unraveling* animations leads to two discoveries: it not only shows how its creative and arbitrary application can be employed to show or hide aspects of the virus, but it also demonstrates its potential to turn the virus into a more or less threatening agent. In fact, the forms and colors chosen for the visualization, as well as the content where this visualization is displayed can evoke very different reactions in the public. Splan extracted four animations from her exercise in spike protein manipulation and colorized them with colors chosen from the software palette which referenced plants, animals, and chemical elements, such as Marine/Aquamarine/Skyblue, Orange/Salmon/Oxygen, Lime/Limon/Forest, and Raspberry/Slate/Violet (McQullan 2020). The resulting animations were

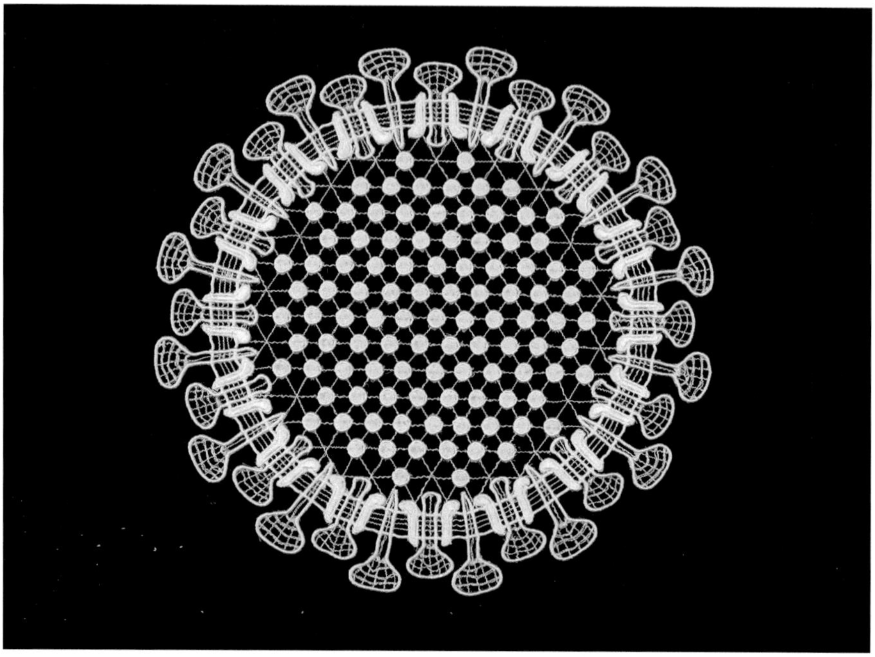

FIGURE 15 *Laura Splan,* Doilies (SARS). © *Laura Splan, 2004.*

displayed on big screens at the Biobat Art Space. Because of the restrictions dictated by the pandemic, the four mandala-like animations could only be accessed by a few visitors at a time: when asked about their experience, a visitor reported that they felt like being in an "electronic womb,[1]" rather than in the presence of a dangerous virus. The virus was not perceived as a threat, as the colors, the meditative experience, and the abstract animation dancing in front of the visitors' eyes widened the distance between them and the virus, temporarily removing them from their apprehensions, perhaps making it less terrifying.

In addition to encouraging the audience to engage in a conversation about the virus, the different forms of representation proposed by Duff, Berrigan and Splan provide clues about its identiti(es), the methodologies that disclose its complexity, and the incredibly tight relationship that the artists have established with it—willingly or by necessity, whether through lab experiment or through software engagement. In these works, the virus emerges as enpresentation; it is made present partially and differently through a combination of scientific procedures and artistic expressions; it is removed from its usual context to evoke new and unconventional experiences.

[1]This specific answer was reported by the artist during an email exchange.

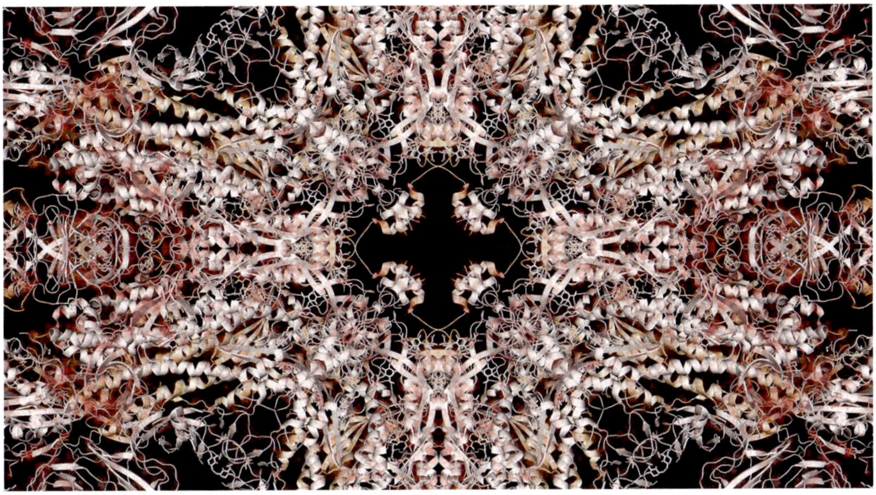

FIGURE 16 *Laura Splan,* Unraveling (Orange/Salmon/Oxygen). © *Laura Splan, 2020. Animation screenshot. Made with PyMOL software. https://www.laurasplan.com/unraveling.*

Layers and Transformation

Duff, Berrigan, and Splan demonstrate how "[v]arious significant relationships exist between the type of referent, the production process, the medium and the types of uses and claims that can be attached to them" (Pauwels 2006, 17). The processes behind visualization can create a safe, and gradually increasing, distance between user and object, viewer and viewed, thus dressing viruses with an appealing and sanitized semblance.

Yet, by doing so, visualization also transcends its object of inquiry. In fact, technologies of display are also technologies of disappearance. Rather than magnifying and sharpening the object of research, they cover it up, hide it underneath countless procedures, digitalization, editing, etc. There is no object to be uncovered, at least not as we figure it, in its "nakedness." The object emerges out of a variety of converging elements and processes every time it becomes visible: it emerges as a bundle of molecules (or bits of code as in the case of computer viruses), as the sum of possible visualizations, and as a symptom. In turn, we as users, researchers, and patients participate in its making and imagine it in its particles, choose how to color it, contribute to its dissemination.

The question we should ask is not what is, or what is left of, the "real object," but, rather, how its multiplicity and the convergence of elements come to form its current visual form and circumstances of display. Interestingly, as the product of techno-cultural relations and one provisional fragment in a sea of processes, viruses come dressed as hybrids that effectively manifest an "implosion of informatics and biologics," one that is "not born, but it is made," as Haraway (1997) so elegantly put it. The virus-turned-object becomes a text dense with metaphors and tropes, a knitted fabric from which we may extract or in which we may see both scientific data and cultural material, and the complex and unavoidable—and often undistinguishable—meshing of information and biology.

The popularity of scientific and data visualizations is in some way a product of the same convergence of culture, aesthetics, models, data, and politics utilized for creating images of biological and computer viruses. When visualizing computer viruses, whose structure and configuration are not directly tied to any physical entity, biological models have served as the basis for the imagined physical form. Although a comparison can be made between the malware that is graphically visualized and the scientific visualizations of biological viruses, the relationship between the two is neither direct nor automatic. The use by computer science of visual elements that are predominantly biological in nature to produce images of computer viruses is a kind of translation. During this process, the object is turned into a record through a "[p]rocess of inscription, transcription, and/or fabrication whereby the initial source (phenomenon or concept) is captured, transformed, or even (re)created through a chain of decisions" (Lynch 2006).

"Despite a surface appearance of unity and rationality," Pauwels argues, "techno-scientific objectification entails far more ambivalence and insecurity, in which closures are performed not by following the rules of scientific method but instead by intuition, symbolic exchange and political association" (Pauwels 2006, 18). Visualizations of malware employ techniques similar to the one used to create scientific visualizations; the object of study is partitioned off from its context and rendered as a geometrical assemblage, consisting of sharp shapes that serve as indicators of their informational nature. The virtual objects, in this case, emerge from both technological translations and cultural models that suggest how computer viruses should look; they draw from a pixel aesthetics that use the classic rendering of real objects on a computer screen, as well as from the numerous metaphors used to describe digitized objects (packets, bits, boxes, etc.). The computer virus is imagined as an assemblage of two-dimensional squares and rectangles.

Visualizing computer viruses has normally been the business of graphic designers and artists—Dragulescu's *Malwarez* series is an example of the works created by such individuals. It should be noted that, while these renditions of popular computer viruses and worms display considerable artistic license, Dragulescu was still compelled to work with programming code in order to faithfully record and render them. The result of a different approach to visualizing viruses, the *Computer Virus Catalogue* consists of renditions of viruses freely interpreted by a designer team commissioned by Amsterdam-based designer Bas van de Poel (Campbell-Dollaghan 2014). In the latter case, the result was a series of illustrations that drew on a different level of significance and set of qualities carried by viruses; rather than trying to reconstruct the appearance of the virus based on its material ontology, the visualizations were based on a combination of the cultural perception and perceived effects of said viruses upon the user.

In September 2005, a 3D animated rendering of the Bagle virus appeared on the F-Secure weblog. This was the first—and probably the last—visual attempt to reproduce dynamically the encounter of a computer virus with its digital host. The animation consisted of a reconstruction of the transformative phases of the computer virus from its initial "dormant" state (i.e., when it is not in contact with any specific host) to its "active" state (i.e., when the user inadvertently triggers the function that will activate the virus). The animation was unique because it mapped the behavior of a computer virus without relying on the stereotypical metaphors and iconic images of death and horror (skulls or other science-fictional references). The animation documented the functions triggered (i.e., the functions enabling the virus to prepare for and perform the attack).

Posted on the F-Secure weblog, and disseminated on popular visualization portals, such as Manuel Lima's visualcomplexity.com (visualcomplexity 2005), this rendering did not reveal any specific feature that would identify the Bagle.AG@mm virus. In fact, the animation could have impersonated any virus. The CBC (Canadian Broadcasting Corporation) incorporated this animation into *Webwarriors*, a feature documentary screened on June 25, 2009, for the series *Doc Zone* (CBC 2009). In this documentary, the animation acquires a CSI-esque significance: the animation appears out of context, as no mention is made of the research merits attached to it. In the documentary, the animation is just another forensic document standing for all computer viruses, an empty signifier merely appearing for theatrical purposes.

The animation represented the final phase of a series of studies to accurately "graph malware." Initially presented at the 2004 Annual Virus Bulletin conference, the first attempt consisted of utilizing the programming functions of a viral agent as reference elements to create a static graphic rendition. This method proposed that viruses should be visualized by reverse engineering their code (Carrera and Erdélyi 2004 and 2004). Carrera and

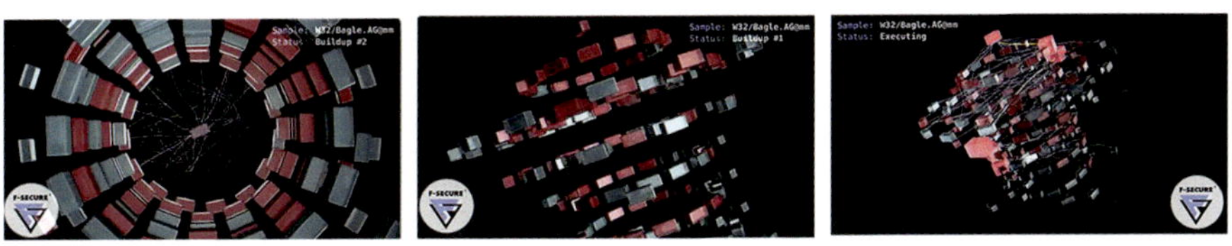

FIGURE 17 *One of the rare animated visualizations of a computer virus: Bagle (F-Secure weblog).*

Erdélyi, two malware analysts at F-Secure, proposed a new visualization method. Focusing on the MyDoom virus, they located and unpacked its functions of and then re-combined them in a two-dimensional visual map. The graphs were obtained by " ... exploring the code of a malware sample looking for all the functions and the relationships between them (who calls who)" (Carrera and Erdélyi 2004, 187).

However, the researchers realized that to gain more insights into the dynamic functioning of the malware, data had to be animated. Visualization would only be partial unless it mapped the various stages of the malware intrusion, including what would trigger the code to call each function and how the execution of the code would unfold. Thus, in the following animation, they processed the same data that had been previously used for the static map, to make them suitable for processing with a 3D software. A special IDA plug-in programmed using Python was employed to prepare the data to be uploaded into the content creation software Blender,[2] so that an animation could be generated.

In Figure 17, the boxes in three pictures stand for functions of the worm all connected and converging at the top, where the execution starts. The virus unfolds through the web of relations formed by its active functions. The animation is useful as it shows the progression of a potential viral attack. According to Axelsson and Sands, this display of data solves a key problem with current intrusion detection systems. With the high amount of daily intrusions, typical network security systems have the tendency to produce many false alarms. Applying information visualization to intrusion detection facilitates the task of recording the progress of viral attacks, and of identifying weaknesses within specific parts of the system (Axelsson and Sands 2006, 80).

The function of the above visual representations and animations to improve the effectiveness of intrusion detection reflects the double drive that dominates visualization: improving knowledge by making the object visible. The object visualized becomes more accessible and manageable. The layers of technology utilized separate the object from the users, allowing them to observe it from a privileged position.

Although the similarity between biological and computer viruses is somehow assumed, in these examples there is also a clear attempt at underscoring their differences. The use of rectangular shapes (as opposed to spherical elements) in the representation of computer viruses makes clear their visual separation from their biological kin and reflects an urge to establish an iconographic precedent in computer virus visualization. By the same token, this new visual paradigm had to take into consideration

[2]Blender is a free, open-source 3D content creation suite, available for all major operating systems under the GNU General Public License. Apparently, this was the best and most convenient option available to the team of researchers: Blender supports Python extensions.

some existing cultural conventions. In order to be recognizable, the representations of computer virus had to reference biological viruses: the allocation of functions that created a spherical, "virus-reminiscent" form catered to this need. The resulting objects reveal the computer virus' functions and active components. At the same time, the virus becomes more distant, as the code now disappears, mediated by layers of processing and visual elements.

As visualization seeks to make viruses more accessible and manageable by turning them into objects that are simultaneously visible and mobile, it also portrays them in isolation, emerging from a sinister darkness granting once again the viewer the position of privileged and protected observer. On the one hand, this format consolidates the idea that viruses (all viruses) are threats appearing from nowhere and poised to damage an unidentified computer or an unaware human host. On the other hand, by isolating the virus, this format separates the potential victim from the virus itself, creating a sense of distance, and therefore of protection.

What seems to be most interesting in this unique series of experiments is the decision to animate the functions of a computer virus. This provides evidence that there is a need to have a more accurate and comprehensive reproduction of the phases that the virus undergoes during its active state. In fact, unlike many other visualizations of biological viruses, which continue to offer static images of a virion, or prefer to create different separate images in order to explicate the transitions of the virus through different states, Carrera and Erdélyi's animation attempts to reproduce the dynamicity of malware (in this case a worm) as it transitions from inactive state to active state.

A similar need had driven artist Tagny Duff in her *Living Viral Tattoo*. Her decision to include both final product (the tattooed skin) as well as the documentation of the process that had led to the product (the laboratory procedures) speaks of a realization that one visual or sculptural product is insufficient when trying to represent a virus. Similarly, Berrigan's multi-part installation emphasizes the different aspects that characterize them: the molecular composition, the epidemiological features, the relation with their human host, etc. Implicit, in all cases, is the awareness that viruses, whether biological or informational, are multifaceted entities that manifest, each time, a different identity.

Beyond the Virus as Object

Given their common mandate to use data to produce visual artifacts, information and scientific visualization intersect at various stages. The reliance on data, and the use of computer-aided techniques to process such data are necessary in the visual construction of both biological and computer viruses. Additionally, the relative novelty of computer-generated visualization[3] calls for lengthy discussions on the nature and aesthetics of visualization. As no strict regulations have been established on how viruses should be represented, the room for creative interpretation increases exponentially, opening the way for a great deal of experimentation.

In all attempts to visualize viruses, scientists and analysts utilize a number of overlapping techniques. In the case of computer viruses, the starting point is just information. But biological viruses are, in the end, also transformed into information. As mentioned in Chapter 3, as soon as the latter are subjected to the electron beams of the microscope, they turn into information and become digitized objects. This phenomenon should make us reflect upon the mediated nature of viruses and the conditions that allow us to see them. If, instead of looking for, or imagining a genuine and pristine object that must be lying underneath these layers, we acknowledge the fact that the images are already hybrid products, created by necessity in order to examine the various aspects of the viruses, would our perception and understanding of viruses change? Would this foster a new awareness regarding the composite and temporary status of these images? Would the refusal to isolate the virus cause our anxiety about viruses to intensify?

If we were to recognize the constructed quality of the images that we consume, and further recognize that they are the products of technology, human intervention, and professional expertise, we would most probably see the resulting objects as things that are neither lost nor hidden, but simply as entities that are always already transformed. The recognition of the process of transformation, as Anna Munster once theorized, is a sign of the decline of Cartesianism and the rise of a new era of the "baroque," that is, an era where the digital loosens its perceived linearity to follow a more elaborate, interconnected, and complicated trajectory. The digital conceived as part of a flow unfolds genealogically out of an articulation of the differential relations between embodiment and technics. In this baroque unfolding, the binary pairs that have populated the understanding of digital culture and new media technologies can be seen to impinge upon each other rather than be mutually exclusive (Munster 2006, 41).

This process of unfolding is already embedded in the processes and mechanisms devised to provide a visual appearance of viruses. What we don't have is the ability to acknowledge it in the media we use to present viruses in their constantly unfinished mediated-ness and in their complexity to larger audiences. Duff and Berrigan, in their installations, demonstrate how this complexity cannot emerge from current visual methods, unless multiple samples are located side by side. The researchers at F-Secure experienced a

[3]According to SIGGRAPH, a leading conference in computer graphics, the "recent emphasis on visualization started in 1987 with the special issue of *Computer Graphics*, [MCCO87], on visualization in scientific computing" (Siggraph 1999).

similar frustration when they realized that a static image could not portray the dynamics and functions of Bagle properly.

The ubiquitous yet ephemeral presence of viruses resonates with Tagny Duff's perspective. Her *Living Viral Tattoos* (Duff 2009) shows us a virus that blends and bleeds, an entity that lives beyond its given boundaries, and constantly exceeds the expectations of the scientist, the artist, or the lay person. The virus is simultaneously alive and undead, multiple and unrepresentable by traditional methods (Duff et al. 2011). The struggle to figure and single out viruses, to even find the appropriate words to speak about them, expresses a conceptual failure, both pertaining to a lack of knowledge of the virus and to an inability to conceive of an entity that seems to escape any attempt to grasp it in its entirety. Berrigan's relation with hepatitis C is intimate and personal, but this personal relationship cannot be translated into scientific parlance.

According to Stephen Ornes, no matter how much information goes into an iconic image of a virus, the result is always to create distance between the virus and the deadly havoc it causes. Whether this reflects a drive to separate and protect the host from the virus, or is a sign that "science is on top of things," it has a major element missing: the image does not resonate with personal experience, or as Rossi maintains, "it is not showing the human side" (Rossi in Ornes 2021). Duff and Berrigan's artworks emphasize two important aspects: the technical and conceptual difficulties related to identifying and communicating the dynamic nature and the pervasiveness of viruses, and the troubles in evaluating and "speaking" their affective import, when epidemics and viral infections appear to hit different individuals in dissimilar ways. Their works expose the partial and often incomplete renditions of the structure and materiality of viruses, that is, their virological aspects, and propose a different way, based on the multiple and the multifaceted, to look at them.

These are important elements that distinguish and complicate viruses. Their heterogeneous and partially unpredictable intertwining with the human and the natural world demonstrates how viruses not only affect, but also are affected by, the individual, the collective, the media, etc. This also brings us to think of the virus as an agent with an epidemiological footprint, rather than just as an object.

5

Situated Epidemiologies

In the previous chapters, I have noted how viruses tend to be presented as well-defined entities; the maintenance of this mode of representation is sustained through technologies and socio-cultural practices. But viruses are not just about their inner structure, their infectious charge, or their appearance. They are also about their spread across human and non-human networks, their behavioral patterns, and the way they can be predicted and contained. They are about the different narratives they generate as well as those that are assigned to them. They are about the way they affect communities, and how such impact exposes more than health.

In this chapter, I examine viral "epidemiologies." Given viruses' multiple vectors of diffusion and impact, I like to refer to epidemiologies in the plural. Because of the complex circumstances and relations that underpin emerging and already circulating viruses, epidemiological research creates projections and hypotheses that may not always reveal the trajectory of viruses or may not always be able to predict their behavior. Pushed by extensive physical, media, and communication networks, patterns of contagion circulate by means of collective and personal narratives, biological exchanges and digital interactions, emotional and social responses.

I will focus on two important technical tools of epidemiological research: epidemiological maps and mathematical models. Like molecular models and illustrations of viruses, maps and models have enjoyed increasing popularity. Their data-driven content grants them an unprecedented authority and power of persuasion (Griffin 2020). Yet, the complexity that characterizes the subjects they study undermines some of their perceived infallibility (Murty 2021). In fact, their design reflects the mandate of the discipline of epidemiology to identify general trends among a population, at the expense of so-called anomalies (Shostak 2010). However, dismissing these very anomalies means neglecting to acknowledge small groups and communities as well as vulnerable or marginalized individuals. Popular maps and models often represent dominant discourses about viruses and viral phenomena, thus suppressing minor narratives. Narratives, collective and personal, coexist in the epidemiological discourse. I am interested in how repetitions, recurring tropes, and other narratives form an "evolving story of disease." Priscilla Wald defined them "outbreak narratives." I want to question the idea of the collective "we," produced by these narratives, and how they permeate the social perception of viral incidents. Biosociality and social solidarity can simultaneously protract homogenizing narratives, creating perceived and material exclusion and isolation, or conversely make space for inclusivity and care.

In this chapter, I reflect on how the display and communication of viral data by means of epidemiological maps and models may lead to the creation, the strengthening, or the challenging of narratives shaping infections and outbreaks. My emphasis will not lie on the accuracy of epidemiological maps and projections, but on the stories they produce and communicate. More specifically, in examining the maps and mathematical projections about outbreaks occurring in computer networks and in the real world, I reflect on the collective narratives they generate. What do they prioritize and what population do they speak to? What/who do they miss and how can artistic work function as a reminder of these absences?

The interdisciplinary project *Visualizing the Virus* initiated by Sria Chatterjee asks these questions. While the project is technically not a map, it acts as a conceptual one, by presenting a kaleidoscopic collection of the many ways SARS-Cov2 (the virus) is being visualized—both by science and by different communities—and how it is perceived through different narratives. Its goal is to expose the inequalities that the virus has suddenly made visible with its passing, by naming the hierarchies and the exclusions that COVID-19 (the disease) has produced. These are all aspects that conventional maps and models are currently unable to underscore. Similarly, Anna Dumitriu's recent pandemic *Ex-Voto* installation features stories of individuals who had personal encounters with the disease. Epidemiological data cannot seize the uniqueness of these stories by design. Similarly, members of the medical profession are unfortunately often forced to ignore them, either because they are considered anecdotal or because the medical field is too overwhelmed and understaffed to acknowledge them. While Dumitriu illuminates personal stories, Ruth Cuthand's series *Trading and Surviving* reclaims recurring symbols of the pandemic to create an alternative narrative that, this time, gives voice to her ancestors.

Epidemiology and the Collection of Data

Epidemiology is the discipline that studies the incidence, the recurrence, and the prediction of given diseases among the population. Epidemiology observes ".. concatenations of biopolitical events that occur within space-time" (Cohen 2011, 17), classifying them according to their frequency and intensity over one or more samples of the population, and proposing lines of intervention and prevention based on their potentials (Rothman 2002; Webb 2005).

Epidemiologists are aware that the spread of epidemics is caused by a considerable number of factors, including the presence of human hosts with different immune systems and medical histories and cultures, environmental conditions, etc. The viral "returns measure to the aesthetic in that aesthetic measure is singular, a measure that changes its metric or perspective with each measure or modulation" (Clough and Puar 2012). In other words, it is a dynamic non-form whose trajectory changes with circumstances; it mutates when in contact with media, histories, and personal accounts. This quality, the viral, makes viruses only partially determinable, as they constantly escape any attempt to anchor them to a definite form or computational figure (Blas 2012). Nonetheless, epidemiology weaves spatio-temporal dimensions together, using reference points such as maps and visual representation to "ground" its findings to a territory, presenting predictions as authoritative and reliable sources of information.

It can be challenging to keep track of multiple outbreaks, especially when they end up becoming full-blown pandemics, and when their spread is not limited to the exclusive relation between the virus and the host but involves and affects entire socio-cultural structures and economic/trade systems. Viral data are collected and processed using mathematical models and laid on maps. While the first usually involve a set of variables and take the visual form of relatively minimal charts (such as line charts, which display data development historically), data employed for epidemic maps are geolocated. The most recent interactive or real-time maps use multiple datasets gathered from different sources, visualized with the assistance of analytics applications such as ArcGIS, Mapbox, Google Maps, among others. Given the goals of epidemiology, its current reliance on big data and digital processing, as well as the constant metaphorical and material link between biological and computer viral outbreaks, techniques of mapping and modeling have been applied successfully and interchangeably to both domains.

Laying data on a map using Geographic Information Systems (GIS) includes "online real-or near-real-time mapping of disease cases and of social media reactions to disease spread, predictive risk mapping using population travel data, and tracing and mapping super-spreader trajectories and contacts across space and time" (Kamel Boulos and Geraghty, 2020). These methods can help speed up the initial detection and characterization of infections. Putting it all together in a mathematical model helps anticipate future infectious disease spread and encourages the adoption of mitigation strategies to contain a potential or already existing epidemic. The two practices are complementary.

According to Tom Koch, managing outbreaks and entire pandemics is a delicate business: "where diagrams, charts, and tables distill and summarize a set of data, mapping as a medium of knowledge assemblage and exploration places that distillation in a context that is at once communal, ecological, and multifactorial" (Koch 2011, 5). It implies considering many variables, such as human and non-human mobility, their social behaviors, land use, origins and phylogenesis and many unknowns, such as population behavior under duress, or unexpected immune responses by different individuals. Although maps and mathematical models offer different ways of examining diseases and outbreaks, they require from the maker and its public a relatively firm trust in the datasets they use. In fact, since maps and models are mostly built thanks to data gathered through semi-automated processes, they are often perceived as neutral and impersonal, and therefore more reliable. This of course doesn't mean that map makers and modelers believe in the infallibility of data. On the contrary, they know that their products contain many unknowns and tentative conclusions. However, they align with the idea that quantitative data can provide the most objective and neutral view on any phenomenon (D'Ignazio and Klein 2020b).

The reluctance of map makers and modelers to present "uncertainty information"—that is, "uncertainty associated with particular pieces of information [which may] help the map reader to answer the question of how much trust to put in that information" (Griffin 2020)—is perhaps caused by this belief. In fact, the fluctuation of results (especially when pandemic conditions are quickly changing) causes maps and projections to deal with various degrees of uncertainty, which are never (or rarely) made explicit when they are made public or when the maps that accompany them are designed. This may create expectations and disappointments, trust and suspicion, whose degree varies from individual to individual, from experience to experience, from circumstance to circumstance.

In epidemiology, the focus is never on the personal aspects of epidemics or the unique ways that viruses may affect individuals—all elements that can complicate the representation of data on a map, or the prediction of coming epidemics. It focuses its attention on entire—or clusters of—communities, creating a comprehensive map of general trends where the focus is on the spread, rather than on the individual, and generates a ".. number of categories of people at risk ... and new opportunities for biomedical surveillance and intervention, self-monitoring, and regimes of behavior change" (Shostak 2010). Mathematical models, statistics, and geo surveillance methods are applied to entire communities, where physical differences, personal and family histories, or individual behavior don't seem to matter, unless they affect the data gathered in significant ways. This practice continues despite growing evidence that current diffusion models often end up being somehow disturbed by myriad other factors (like environmental, cultural, and social factors) that contribute to the changing of the trajectory and the formation of any pandemic (Cepelewicz 2021; Grubaugh et al. 2019). By maintaining a general view on populations and on general trends, epidemiological maps and modeling rely on principles founded in biopolitics (Rose 2001; Shostak 2010).

Epistemic Uncertainty

In *The Birth of the Clinic,* Michel Foucault explained how epidemiology, founded in the eighteenth century, seeks to detect recursive signs that medical practitioners can use to describe generalized trends within specific medical episodes (Foucault 1994). According to Foucault, epidemics are simultaneously general and particular, since they do not have "a sort of historical individuality, hence the need to employ a complex method of observation when dealing with [them]," yet, as collective phenomena they "require a multiple gaze" and "must be described in terms of [their] special, accidental, unexpected qualities" (22). This quality complicates the study and identification of general trends: trends always take on different meanings, they cause different reactions, and they evoke different feelings in different contexts from different individuals. However, the researcher must look for recursive events and repetitions, in order to categorize them and be able to study and anticipate the coming of new epidemics.

This approach does not leave any room for uncertainty. Although the mapping and monitoring of epidemics change over time, including new variables, these elements are never made explicit when presented officially. In addition, because of the complexity of such phenomena, no matter how much data is gathered and processed, mapping and modeling outbreaks will never produce exact results (Grubaugh et al. 2019). Furthermore, Griffin explains (2020), "although the benefit of helping public health decision makers understand the limitations of mapped data is clear, perhaps some mapmakers believe that the public will not understand data uncertainty" (13).

The same problem occurs with modeling. It is believed that providing uncertainty data may be damaging to public communication as it creates ambiguities and potential problems of trust, despite evidence that "people have a positive reaction and trust information more when the communicator is being open about uncertainties in facts and figures" (Roberts 2020a). Siobhan Roberts refers to the general "uncertainty about facts, numbers and science" that we are experiencing today with the pandemic as epistemic uncertainty (ibid.). Navigating a sea of unknowns and dealing with unexpected outcomes is how science has always functioned and is at the center of the experimental practice. However, scientists may be reluctant to publicly admit to the inherent uncertainties that prevent them from giving exact solutions. Many fear that being honest will discredit their work, falling again for the belief that science, and its quantified rigor, will provide the right answer. Roberts suggests that admitting the imperfection of science in general, and mathematical models in particular, may create a healthier relationship between the public and science.

Epidemiology prioritizes quantitative evidence over qualitative judgment. This preference is in part epistemological and applies to maps and models equally; Lisa Cartwright explains that "the qualitative and empirical gaze of the eighteenth and the nineteenth century anatomo-clinical perception … overlapped with and was ultimately challenged by the relentlessly analytical and quantitative gaze … a mode of perception carefully incubated within the laboratories of physiologists and medical scientists" (Cartwright 1995, xiii). Nicholas Rose ascribes this prioritizing of data to the rise of risk thinking, which calculates "probable futures in the present followed by interventions into the present in order to control a potential future" (Rose 2001, 11). Methods based on statistics and probabilistic reasoning have "trust in numbers" replacing "other forms of trust" (13).

José Van Djick and Lisa Cartwright suggest that in addition to probabilistic reasoning, increasing technological development has played a crucial role in gradually substituting "direct sensory perception" with protocols, to the extent that innovation has become the result of a constant "attunement of machines and bodies, of procedures and images, of interpretations and protocols" (van Dijck 2005, 7). Perhaps this is not surprising, considering that advanced technologies have allowed human beings to achieve things that would be difficult or impossible if we had to rely solely on our unaided senses or intellectual abilities. For instance, new data-mining techniques and the digitization of many scientific procedures have made it possible to capture details about phenomena that might otherwise have been undetectable. Technologies have lent great versatility to epidemiological research: new software has also enabled scientists to examine, package, and communicate epidemiological data in immediate visual forms (Friendly 2008). The specific qualities of the digital (mainly their scalability, variability, and partial numerical automation, as described by Lev Manovich in his 2001 book) have empowered scientists to process increasingly voluminous amounts of data.

The rise of big data has produced a new confidence in the mechanisms and technologies of mapping and visualization, and their claims to be able to measure, rank, and classify all aspects of the world in precise and allegedly objective, not to mention, aesthetically stunning ways (Dalton, Taylor, and Thatcher 2016; Thatcher 2014). Unsurprisingly, many scientists and clinicians have welcomed its emergence with much enthusiasm, as they see in big data's ability to collect and represent increasingly large sets of data using semi-automatic digitization processes a remarkable opportunity (Murdoch and Detsky 2013, for instance, spoke of the application of big data in health care as an inevitable step).

Despite the sophistication of the technologies available, it is important to keep in mind that pathogens, malware, and the geographical/network territory they affect, its population, and its surrounding conditions, are all elements whose parameters mutate relatively quickly. With multiple factors colliding and intertwining, it becomes difficult to predict with certainty the spread of outbreaks and to contain individuals' behaviors and mobility. This was demonstrated throughout the 2020 coronavirus pandemic, where epidemiological projections were often exaggerating, or unable to fully predict the pandemic outcomes, because of the lack of data and because of the role that unexpected or unaccounted factors played in changing the course of the disease (Brossard and Lewenstein 2010; Cepelewicz 2021). In mapping outbreaks, maps may show different results, because data are aggregated from different sources, are laid by means of different styles, or simply present different perspectives (Griffin 2020).

It is currently not possible to predict with absolute precision the trajectory of viral infections. This is not only because too many factors contribute to shaping such trajectories. It is also because the people affected by viral outbreaks are often counted just as "variables" or as "quantifiable categories." Epidemiology does not and cannot account for the way different individuals react to a given infectious condition, and the way this condition affects different people in different ways.

Mapping Worldwide Diseases: People as "Blobs"

There are similarities and overlapping between the way that infectious diseases and malware are mapped: for Laszlo Barabási, if the circulation of infections can be mapped (and thus anticipated) by focusing on the nodes that infectious diseases cross and into which they converge during their journey, then not only is it not necessary to analyze the entire network of contagion, but it is also possible to avoid following specific carriers of disease and, rather, investigate "safer traveling objects" (Barabási 2003). In other words, in order to identify the impact of an outbreak, rather than focusing on the individual entity causing the epidemic, one can look at the objects (or organisms) that may likely transport it. Danon et al. confirm that there exists an "extremely close relationship between epidemiology and network theory ... This is because the connections between individuals (or groups of individuals) that allow an infectious disease to propagate naturally define a network, while the network that is generated provides insights into the epidemiological dynamics" (Danon et al. 2011). Four forms of "movement network" have played important roles in understanding the spread of infectious diseases: Danon et al., for instance, list the airline transportation network, the movement of individuals to and from work, the movement of dollar bills (from which the movement of people can be inferred), and the movement of livestock (especially cattle). As a matter of fact, the earliest work using detailed movement data to drive simulations comes from the spread of the 1918 pandemic influenza in the Canadian Subarctic, data that were based on records kept by the Hudson's Bay Company (Dimka 2015; Sattenspiel and Herring 1998).

Mark Monmonier observes that while "Reality is three-dimensional, rich in detail, and far too factual to allow a complete yet uncluttered two-dimensional graphic scale model … a map that did not generalize would be useless" (Monmonier 1996, 25). Both malware maps and infectious disease maps reproduce the territory to be examined in a simplified format, which allows researchers to not only better examine an epidemic incident, find anomalies, or map the progression of a disease, but also to better communicate with a range of different audiences, including epidemiologists, medical doctors, emergency doctors, security analysts, etc.

Mapping and visualization allow us to zoom in and inspect certain objects or areas of research more closely. They can also help us zoom out to take in a general trend, providing a birds-eye view of a given phenomenon, or an epidemiological study. One may recall the classic epidemic maps popularized in the nineteenth century by John Snow (Koch 2011). These maps famously facilitated impressive breakthroughs in the understanding of localized epidemic outbreaks (in this case an outbreak of cholera in London) and were instrumental in investigating their cause.

There exist many epidemiological maps displaying infectious and emerging diseases (Ebola, SARS-CoV-2, MERS, etc.), socially determined conditions (diabetes, obesity, malnutrition, etc.), or the spread of one or several network threats. Because of the spread of cyber threats across the world at any given time, maps usually display real time dynamic data. In recent maps, real-time data are represented as fast streams of light speeding from point A to point B, color-coded differently according to the type of threat they represent. This is very different from the way malware was displayed only a few years ago, when the focus was only on a few particularly threatening worms and Trojan horses with exotic names.

Most of the cybersecurity maps are produced by security companies such as Kaspersky Lab. Historically, these maps have displayed many similarities with the surveillance methods used by the Centers for Disease Control and Prevention and the World Health Organization used to monitor the emergence of flu and other novel diseases. In fact, their color-coded warning was modeled after the one conventionally utilized to measure the national security status (from green to red) in the United States. Their goals were epidemiology-inspired: to identify concentrations of multiple threats and their trajectory, to determine which area should be more intensely monitored. While they provided a clear and ordered picture of some viral activity, only a few viruses and worms—usually those causing most concern—were displayed. Each antivirus company arbitrarily decided which viral threat to feature, based on their judgment of the danger posed by a virus. For instance, if the company was specialized in the detection of mobile phone security vulnerabilities, the map would feature these threats. The degree of danger was measured according to the mandate of the company.

The tone of urgency of the early maps has decreased substantially in recent years. When comparing maps disseminated in the early 2000s to today's maps, one may find that their design and narrative have become closer to a game than to an epidemiological map. Some maps even come with demo

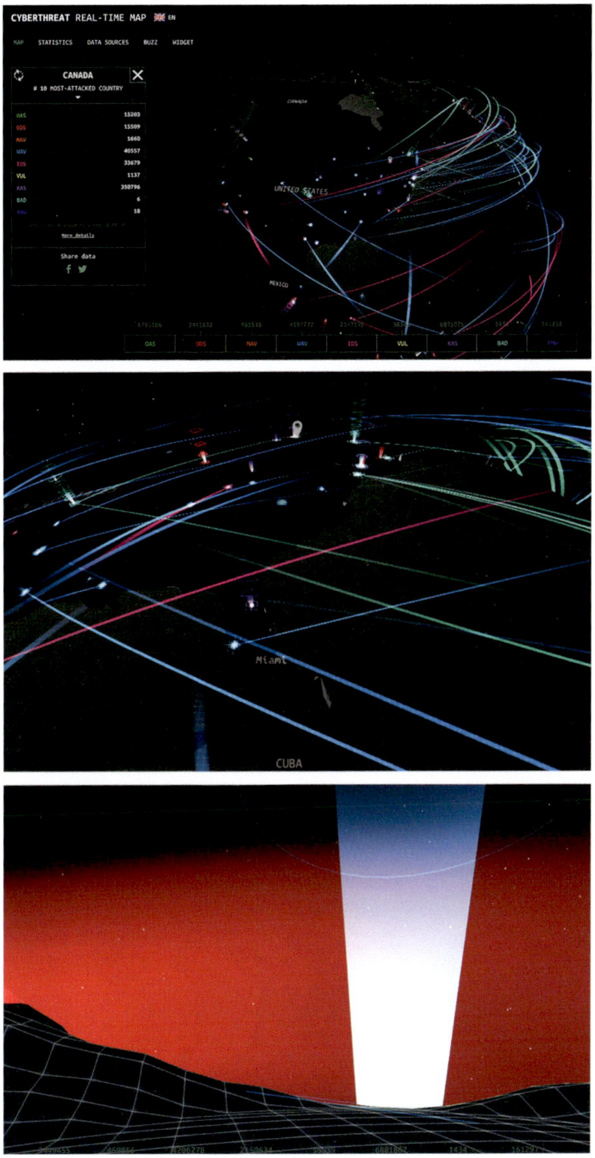

FIGURE 18 Cyberthreat Real-Time Map *by Kaspersky Lab. https://cybermap.kaspersky.com/ for different views. The viewer can zoom in and explore specific categories of malware or vulnerabilities, or let the map switch to closeups and 3D animations in demo mode.*

mode, displaying appealing and colorful 3D animations. This is the case of the Kaspersky Lab's real-time map (Figure 18) (Kaspersky Lab n.d.). The differentiation of malware may have triggered the quasi-gamification of these maps. The intensification of online activity, as well as the increasing popularity of mobile devices—the iPhone is famously considered crucial to the expansion of social media and app culture, as well as network mobility (Burgess 2012)—and the ubiquity of Internet of Things (IoT) devices have caused security threats to diversify and adapt to a range of different technologies. Before the rise in popularity of these technologies, computer viruses, worms, and Trojan horses used to be the most urgent, pervasive, and serious threats to networks security and network privacy. Single worms with memorable names like ILoveYou or MyDoom threatening entire network clusters have become rarer (or more manageable) and have been replaced by phishing attacks, ransomware, and other different—yet equally insidious—threats.

Displaying such growing diversity on a map has become not only more challenging, but also irrelevant. Thus, today's maps display categories—such as "ransomware" or "vulnerability," etc.— rather than single threats, and prioritize trends and flows rather than single worms or viruses. While the color-coded signals are still used, they no longer scream danger, as bright red, orange, and yellow are substituted by faint red, baby blue, pastel pink, and fuchsia. The diversification and specialization of cyber threats have also made the mimicking of CDC and WHO obsolete since the comparison of current cybersecurity risks to a flu or an infectious disease no longer holds. Finally, the rise of emerging infectious diseases in the face of climate change and, recently, a global pandemic, has seen a rapid intensification of interest in infectious disease maps, turning the mapping of such threats THE most popular form of epidemiological mapping.

Among the many infectious disease maps monitoring the spread of the SARS-CoV-2 virus, the Johns Hopkins University map and dashboard stands out as one of the most popular. Created by Lauren Gardner and then graduate student Ensheng Dong at the Centre for System Science and Engineering, the map was developed to "provide researchers, public health authorities, and the general public with a user-friendly tool to track the outbreak as it unfolds," and aggregated data from several sources and locations (Coronavirus Resource Centre 2020).[1]

Griffin suggests that a probable source of popularity of this map was its promptness as it was one of the first maps of COVID-19 to be published. However, it reached more popularity than other maps that appeared almost simultaneously, like the WHO map, because ".. at least to Western eyes, its color choices connote danger and urgency: a black background and saturated red symbols" (Griffin 2020). Other maps sported a terser, less threatening set of colors (WHO's different shades of blue or a range of different colors).

[1]"The data sources include the World Health Organization, the US Centers for Disease Control and Prevention, the European Center for Disease Prevention and Control, the National Health Commission of the People's Republic of China, 1point3acres, Worldometers.info, BNO, state and national government health departments, local media reports, and the DXY, one of the world's largest online communities for physicians, health care professionals, pharmacies and facilities" (Coronavirus Resource Centre 2020).

The Johns Hopkins map and shown in Figure 19 first appeared in January 22, 2020, when it was clear that what appeared to be an anomalous pneumonia was indeed a new infectious disease caused by a novel coronavirus (Dong et al. 2020). The map has not only become a go-to resource, but it has also succeeded in conveying the appropriate urgency of the situation: it relentlessly updates its numbers with rhythmic precision, automatically retrieving them from various datasets, and classifying them by infection cases, mortality rates, and, more recently, by vaccination numbers. Data appear on a simple black and gray map of the world map as red blobs, their circumferences expanding with increased infections in quasi real time. The authors of the map chose to display the outbreaks using red, the color of terror, fear, and the color of maximum alert used in many earlier disease and cybersecurity maps, as well as the color assigned to highest national security danger in the United States and many other countries.

The appearance of the expanding red dots almost filling the map, accompanied by the unstoppable pace of the numbers of deaths and infections, created a dramatic outlook that did more than just provide information. Observing the pandemic occupying larger geographical areas did provide information about its course, leaving a sense of urgency and growing powerlessness. In a way, this early map stood as a hyperreal show, one reminiscent of the sequences of chilling strike precision that had inundated international TV news during the two Iraqi Wars in the 1990s and early 2000s. The latter presented a spectacle of horror packaged as a morbid video game, a vision that made people doubt that such a faraway war, as Jean Baudrilland (Baudrillard 1995) noted, was not even taking place, disappeared, as it was, in the haze of media distance.

The Johns Hopkins map is successful in evoking concerns. However, like most maps with such a focused goal, it does not provide any information about different patterns of contagion, reactions to the pandemic, or local actions to mitigate it. It doesn't attempt to answer questions such as why were some countries more severely affected than others, while other countries seemed to do much better? Was it because of the carelessness or rule-breaking behavior of certain countries, their aging population, their environment? How did age and family compositions, population density and industrial concentration, cultural habits, environmental factors, and different governance systems affect the course of the pandemic (Tufekci 2020)?

The Johns Hopkins map evokes emotions in the reader but treats the subjects it portrays emotionlessly. All incidents are equal and no specific information is provided about the different ways the virus affected/infected a population. Of course the goal of the map is not to provide information about individual experiences, but to give a general sense of the gravity of the situation worldwide. To do this, the mapmakers had no choice but to turn people into red blobs and numerical values.

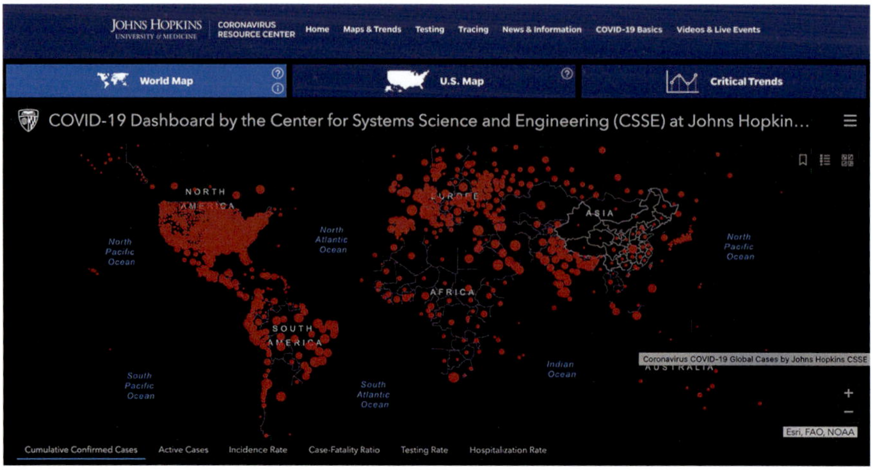

FIGURE 19 *COVID-19 map FAQ, 2020. Johns Hopkins Coronavirus Resource Center. Map of active cases, recovered and deaths by country. Accessed July 14, 2020. https://coronavirus.jhu.edu.*

Trust the Numbers? Mathematical Modeling and the Problem of Uncertainty

Quantitative data and geospatial datasets are generally considered more trustworthy than qualitative analyses, even when the information contained in the dataset used is not entirely reliable (Griffin 2020). A similar trust is placed in mathematical models. During the coronavirus pandemic, mathematical models have registered a certain increase in popularity for their potential to partially predict its spread and flesh out the role of human behavior in its expansion.

In the classic SIR model (or compartmental model) and its variations, the arc of a pandemic is based on three types of populations: the Susceptible (the individual who could contract the virus), the Infectious (the already-infected individual informing the rate of spread), and the Recovered (the one who is no longer contributing to the spread, because vaccinated or dead). The more variables are introduced, the more complex the model becomes. For instance, in the agent-based or individual spread model, the individuals' infectivity and exposure depend on whether they infect family, colleagues, people they meet in public, or during other random occasions (Hoertel et al. 2020). When people are represented in a network model, individuals are treated according to graph theory, that is, instead of being "hosts" and "contacts," or "actors" and "relations," they become nodes and edges in a complicated lattice: "In each case, it is the presence of a relationship between individuals in a population that is the issue of concern" (Keeling and Eames 2005).

Policymakers found mathematical models especially useful. They turned to modelers to help them make decisions about reopening businesses and schools after an outbreak, or about adopting or relaxing safety measures during the receding of a pandemic (Cepelewicz 2021). Epidemiologists and modelers are well aware of the inability of models to provide complete and accurate predictions. Adam Kucharski argues that a model "is just a way of understanding a particular process or a particular question we're interested in. The point is to understand what is the trend, what is the qualitative take-home message you get from this" (Cepelewicz 2021). Kumar Murty warns that models " ... are not perfect because they are designed to fit a particular epistemology, and they are not perfect because the spirit of science is not about exactitude but experimentation" (Murty 2021). These positions are not uncommon among the mathematics and modeling community. Famously, as statistician George Box pointed out, "all models are wrong, but some are useful": it is not the exact result that counts the most in a model, but how useful it is to help understand a phenomenon (Box 1976). However, when models emerge in the public domain and become instrumental in making important life-saving policy decisions, it is their quantitative content, not their qualitative usefulness that is most valued. When they go public, models are (and must be) presented as reliable. Then, when reality does not match the predictions, criticisms turn into complete lack of trust (Buiani 2021; Holmdahl and Buckee 2020; Tufekci 2020).

The deep sense of uncertainty that the coronavirus pandemic precipitated put an unfair pressure on the model as a reliable tool. Its self-imposed confidence created an initial degree of comfort until—like everything else in the pandemic—it turned into something that can't provide indisputable answers and clear guidelines. Modeling, although useful, is then seen as a failure because it does not perform as expected. This leads to counterproductive reactions.

There is no doubt that instrumentalization and politics, on the one hand, and scientific illiteracy on the other play major roles in creating a discrepancy between what models do and how they are presented and perceived. However, this very discrepancy also signals an epistemic tendency to overemphasize the role of quantification in solving a problem that is naturally complex. Realizing that quantified content is not effective in tackling such complex an issue may lead to an intensification of the general sense of uncertainty that has already dominated the current situation. When this discrepancy becomes exposed, it reveals how current beliefs and assumptions about scientific reliability are caused by many juxtaposing factors, not just by whether or not a model is correct. In fact, these factors are all equally contributing to fueling or dissipating uncertainty. In the case of the 2020 pandemic, analyzing this discrepancy could have suggested a few long-term strategies to address, acknowledge, and communicate its inherent complexity and its stochastic qualities.

It is important to remember that models, although sometimes very accurate—especially when they contain a big number of historical data—are simulations. They propose a "what if" scenario based on what is currently known. Not unlike bacteria studied in a controlled environment such as a Petri dish, a population is evaluated according to a set of established—though constantly growing and diversifying—parameters. Even when these parameters are fed into an AI system, many unknowns are unavoidably left uncovered. Models "simplify a human population into a series of groups, or compartments, across which individuals move as a function of their epidemic status, age, or position in the social network: susceptible, infectious, exposed, asymptomatic, those who recover, those who die, those at high risk of exposure, and those most likely to infect others" (Poisot 2020). In fact, models are not just there to make exact predictions, but to persuade, especially during circumstances such as a pandemic (O'Neil 2020a), where the resulting predictions are meant to convince a school or a government to pass new regulations, to modify one's behavior to suit, or to change course from, the prediction.

This is what happened in mid-March 2020 during the early phase of the SARS-CoV-2 pandemic when a research team at Imperial College London used an agent-based model to convince governments that refusing to implement any form of quarantine would have disastrous consequences. Its projection predicted up to half a million deaths from COVID-19 in the UK alone, and 2.2 million deaths in the United States if nothing was done to mitigate the spread (Ferguson et al. 2020, 9). The model was not supposed to provide exact numbers, but to persuade policymakers to act urgently (Cepelewicz 2021). As a result, British Prime Minister Boris Johnson almost immediately announced stringent new restrictions on people's movements. The United States announced social distancing rules soon after (Adam 2020). Similarly, in 2021, models released by the Ontario COVID-19 Science Advisory Table were used to prolong the lockdown in specific areas of the province most severely hit by the B.1.1.7. variant of concern (now known as Alpha, CBC News 2021).

Policymakers and governments maintain a relative trust in models. Of course, until they fail. Trust quickly turns into criticism when the numbers predicted by these models look inflated or don't match the expectations. For quantitative epidemiologist Matthew Ferrari, when an unrealistic projection is consciously published and later proved wrong, we should not consider it a failure. Quite the opposite: "The best early models are the ones that are wrong, precisely because we react to them and make them wrong". If the projection was proved right, it would mean that it has failed to persuade (Cepelewicz 2021, accompanying video). Models like the one produced at the Imperial College were picturing a purposely exaggerated doomsday scenario. Because governments took precautions, cases and death ended up less numerous than expected.

Outcomes do not always turn out better than expected. When the projections produce unexpected negative outcomes, criticism leads to mistrust or outright rejection of the modeling practice, threatening its value and its validity. The unfortunate failure of the model created at the University of Illinois at Urbana-Champaign (UIUC) is a case in point. In order to preserve the safety of students and staff as they were returning to campus, physicists Nigel Goldenfeld, Sergei Maslov, and their research team created a network-based predictive model which they complemented with frequent COVID-19 tests and—they assumed—strict surveillance strategies. The main purpose of the model was not to make precise predictions, but to help administrators make informed choices on the best way to allow classes and other activities to resume safely and smoothly (Chang 2020). The result was a massive and expensive operation: 40,000 students were asked to take specially designed fast-diagnostics saliva tests twice a week (the university paid $10 for each test). In addition, students had to register for a contact tracing app: if their test turned positive, they would lose access to the university buildings and would have to be confined to their dorms. The model had even introduced a variable anticipating that more than 7,000 students would go partying three times a week, despite the current social distancing restrictions (Nadwordny 2020).

However, mere weeks after the opening of the campus, it became clear that the model had failed. In trying to contemplate all the possible variables, the two scholars and their interdisciplinary team had assumed that students would follow the recommendations established by the university administration. Even though they knew that the students are notorious for breaking rules, they did not anticipate that several of them would continue to go to parties even after testing positive. Some of these students even "tried to circumvent the app so that they could enter buildings instead of staying isolated in their rooms" (Chang 2020).

As a result, the model was not able to predict the speed at which (infected) students would spread the disease among their (susceptible) peers, compromising the validity of the simulation and leading to dramatic real-life results. Cases immediately grew exponentially, reaching in one week the numbers that had been estimated for months later. Several media outlets and skeptical critics, as well as (and especially) flat-out anti-science politicians read this case as one more reason to mistrust all models and ultimately all scientific projections (Cepelewicz 2021).

From the perspective of the person consulting models and maps, the privilege of being able to follow the unfolding of an epidemic is counterbalanced by an increased anxiety arising from the view of the progression of the infection. A map showing the spread of a disease may produce different results due to the datasets it uses. Similarly, a model may not perform according to expectations. The variables comprising it might show exaggerated data or contain enough small errors to skew its results. Yet, the value that models hold as qualitative guidelines is often ignored. In both cases, maps and models produce a temporary sense of confidence and reassurance from big data and mathematics. At the same time, their inability to perform as expected causes anxiety.

Data and Storytelling

Besides being imperfect, maps and models are phenomenal storytellers. Their narratives evoke responses that are both collective and individual. Collective, because their form and design situate them in a particular socio-cultural context and give behavioral and emotional guidance to the viewer. Individual, because they unavoidably trigger very different personal reactions. Catherine D'Ignazio and Lauren Klein note that persuasion is everywhere, even in spreadsheets (D'Ignazio and Klein 2020). However, for many map makers and data analysts, this is up for debate. For instance, data visualization scholars Alberto Cairo and Edward Tufte claim that the work of professionals who actively shape data should be a curated product of automated processes. Since it is not possible to include all collected data in one map or one, to "curate" means to reduce data clutter and to organize the content in such way that the most essential information is transmitted to the receiver, to deliver a clear message. The maker should let data speak for themselves (Cairo 2016; Tufte 2001). In other words, the maker's role is to make the message more legible. Design and colors should neither make suggestions, nor convey any emotion: "Emotion is often exiled from data science, seen as a suspicious element that may introduce subjectivity into an otherwise 'objective' process" (D'Ignazio and F. Klein 2020).

D'Ignazio and Klein reject the artificially neutral view of maps and graphs: a map or a graph representing the results of a model is never neutral. Donna Haraway famously called this presumed neutral look "the god trick of seeing everything from nowhere" (Haraway 1988). While the red blobs displayed in the Johns Hopkins map are the product of data collection, they follow a specific aesthetic and epistemological choice that is certainly not random. The increasing circumference of the blobs threatening to cover the map at any point, and their chosen color are meant to sound the alarm about the unfolding pandemic and to make people aware of the dangers of the coronavirus. This design has succeeded in capturing the attention of the viewer: Griffin remarks that the Johns Hopkins' map of COVID-19 has worked so well because it is "emotionally arousing, especially in comparison with the rather staid, neutral appearance of the WHO map" (Griffin 2020). The use of less dramatic colors in the latter (mostly shades of blue or purple) improved its authoritative score, because a neutral palette is "typical of the authoritative rhetorical style" (ibid.). However, it did not make it go viral.

The Johns Hopkins map was able to convey an urgent and clear message thanks to a few simple design decisions. When examining the visual history of cyberthreat maps in the past fifteen years, the transformation of design indicates a substantial shift in the perception of cyberthreat. By turning into stylish animated exercises, these maps signal a semantic and rhetorical separation from the typical maps produced by the WHO and the CDC.

They no longer resemble epidemiological maps, indicating that comparing cyberthreats to biological infections might no longer be meaningful or useful. With the main threat no longer being a computer virus or a worm, but an increasing variety of diverse threats with different qualities and gravity, the comparison with the biological has become less evident.

Jason Farman observes that the process of extraction and simplification of the cartographic and data mapping practices suppress "truth to help the user see what needs to be seen" (Farman 2010, 872). What "needs to be seen" for Farman is constituted by a dominant view on the phenomenon mapped, characterized by visual conventions and signs that map makers are obliged to respect, and by narratives that the assumed target public will likely understand. For example, the choice of most mathematical modelers to represent the development of the COVID-19 pandemic on a line graph or time plot is both visually compelling and semiotically telling: in fact, line graphs are excellent at showing data over time and in a continuum. A line graph supplies a single continuous and simple visual item, which communicates instantaneously and intuitively the seriousness of the pandemic. Predilecting this type of graph over histograms or scatter charts is an important move. The infamous "pandemic curve" became a ubiquitous symbol, immortalized in several editorial cartoons and illustrations across the world.

Maps and models produce narratives that tend to reproduce the expectations, the effects, and the fear of infectious diseases. Not only do narratives reflect how societies react to infectious diseases through different forms of storytelling, they also create communities around such diseases (Wald 2008, 3). The narratives disseminated about infectious diseases and pandemics contain recurring patterns that erase individual experience and enhance the experiences of one assumed community or one sector of the population, suggesting how this population should behave in front of a certain experience of the disease, or making assumptions about how the majority of the population reacts to such disease.

Epidemiology searches for data-rich narratives since they can help in its investigations. By describing outbreaks by means of uniform and agreed-upon terms and narration techniques, epidemiologists learn to recognize the patterns of a disease. However, these narratives are quantified; clues are used to diagnose and describe infectious diseases according to patterns, statistics and data about infection rate, demographics, etc. In fact, the translation of a communicable disease into a narrative enables the epidemiologist to focus on "the group, or population, rather than the individual, and tell a story about that group in the language of disease and health" (28). Thus, epidemiological maps and narratives serve both scientific and political goals: they identify a set of behavioral patterns that may be used to successfully speed up the understanding and prompt seizing of a pandemic. At the same time, they guide the reactions to the said pandemic, thus suggesting how the population should face an outbreak.

Biosociality and Outbreak Narratives: Whom Does Collective Behavior Serve?

Epidemics, Ed Cohen observes, are political and biopolitical phenomena, whose containment reveals and confounds "our understanding both of how individuals constitute our collectives and of how we exclude other collectivities that might not belong to them" (Cohen 2011, 15). In fact, epidemiology "relies on and reproduces assumptions about what constitutes a group or a population, about the definition of pathology and well-being and about the connection between disease and 'the lifestyle and behavior of different groups'" (Wald 2008, 19). The double qualitative and quantitative aspects of these narratives facilitate the delineation of the "membership and scale of a population" (Cohen 2011, 20)—that is, its belonging to or its exclusion from a particular group of similarly affected individuals—and creates protocols and standards to assess—quantitatively, that is, by collecting data—an outbreak.

As Michel Foucault points out, the history of "ideas, sciences and knowledge" (Foucault 1989a, 24) is dominated by notions suggesting the existence of " ... ready-made syntheses, [some] groupings that we normally accept before any examination, [links] whose validity is recognized from the outset" (25). The existence of these groupings ensures ".. the infinite [and unquestioned] continuity of discourse and its secret presence *to itself* in the interplay of a constantly recurring presence" (28, emphasis is mine). Foucault questions the uncritical acceptance of given continuities and calls for a "suspension of all accepted unities" (31). These unities should not be discarded as a whole, but analyzed as the "totality of all effective statements in their dispersion as events and in the occurrence that is proper to them" (29). Dispersed statements about viruses follow heterogeneous routes: they not only coagulate into discursive conglomerates outside the constraints of history, disciplinary boundaries, or science, but they also recur and are applied to different circumstances and by different individuals.

Foucault's "groupings" and "unities" remind me of two aspects regarding the way infectious episodes are communicated and perceived. First, coverage of, and information about pandemics, infectious diseases, and network disruptions tend to come to us in fragmented forms and are subject to categorization: virological information and epidemiological data tend to be presented separately; socio-cultural analysis and reflections have no place in a scientific discourse until they are backed by empirical data; artistic, literary, or creative reactions to epidemics are seldom mixed with scientific accounts. When they are, they immediately lose their scientific value, or are classified as art; in certain cases, they become science communication, this time losing their artistic significance. Second, hegemonic narratives and repetitive discourses recur as refrains, and are applied across entire populations as if epidemics evoked the same reactions across one or more populations.

Priscilla Wald called the "evolving story of disease" based on repetitions, recurring tropes and other narrative formulas "outbreak narrative" (Wald 2008). The resulting stories and tropes join beliefs, behaviors, and best practices to avoid contagion and illness. Often, the use of these practices, prompted by unclear or fast changing directives, as well as a certain fatigue to adjust frequently to these directives, becomes indiscriminate or unfocused, to the extent that it ends up obscuring real effective practices and creating a false sense of security. Hygiene practices like washing hands and sanitizing groceries or using masks as a precautionary move belong to a group of collective "beliefs that microbes cause disease and can be avoided by certain protective behavior." This may result in obsessive behavior with counterproductive effects, as in the case of what Nancy Tomes calls "the gospel of germs" (Tomes 1999, 2), or in a total rejection when instructions to maintain such behaviors are confusing, or are not leading to immediate resolutions.

Outbreak narratives evoke a variety of responses to pandemic. But whose voice is it, and whom are they representing? The voice of a collective and homogeneous "we"? According to Wald, the outbreak narratives generated by epidemiological analyses and media coverage of pandemics tend to form homogeneous perceptions of epidemics and infectious diseases, thus making the "route of transmission visible" and helping epidemiologists "anticipate and manage the course of the outbreak" (Wald 2008, 18). This is a top-down approach: scientific authorities (the CDC, WHO, local science tables, and official panels of experts) and the media manage the distribution of these narratives. "When epidemiology turns an outbreak of communicable disease into a narrative," Wald continues, "it makes the route of transmission visible" (19), turning narratives into an instrument not unlike the microscope, a technology that not only creates protocols and standards to assess a phenomenon, but also facilitates the delineation of the "membership and scale of a population" (20).

Outbreak narratives form a network of consensus and affective sharing. On the one hand, these reactions are emotional, both unique and collective (i.e., our personal experience of a disease is not someone else's; repetitive details and narratives mobilize collective reactions). On the other hand, they come in the form of a series of formulas or refrains. They do not indicate any specific infectious episode, yet they can cause serious concerns. These refrains are repetitive and modular, they are both attached to specific infectious episodes, and adapt to more recent ones. They can be found engrained in the socio-cultural context as much as in the scientific tools of retrieval and display.

Thus, the use of outbreak narratives helps identify and delimit the population, which, the narrative tells us, is receiving the pathogen as a—healthy and unadulterated—"we," a pristine "inside" threatened by an evil force coming from the "outside." Besides the immediately visible binary conceptualization putting viruses and humans against each other without mentioning the complex intertwining with other environmental and social factors, these guiding narratives draw direct connections between the advent of an infectious disease and the mistrust toward the other—be this other microbial or animal or human—and unleash, in the case of human "others," racist or cruel assumptions about the culturally diverse. As a result, such narratives have the double role of defining and delimiting a population, implicitly revealing other "tensions that cut across our biopolitical parsing of the world" (Cohen 2011, 16).

Caitlin Berrigan's *How to Befriend a Virus* in Chapter 4 was concerned with a virus—hepatitis C—that the artist herself affirms "lacks any biosociality." In fact, hepatitis C has a "distributed and heterogeneous" and "racially complicated" articulation (Berrigan 2012), affecting a quantitative majority of white men, but a statistically higher portion of African-American men. The virus is transmitted via contact with blood from an infected person: it can be passed through sharing infected needles, transfusions, or even at birth if the mother carries the virus. Not only is there no common narrative that collectively unifies the experiences of those with the disease (like the narratives produced by large outbreaks such as the plague, AIDS, or today's COVID-19 pandemic), but any narrative emerging is also inevitably based on personal and largely isolated stories. The dispersed nature of this disease has left many affected individuals to deal with this condition on their own. This, according to Berrigan, is a problem as the individuals suffering from the condition have little ability to share their experiences.

Biosociality is the tendency of individuals to base their social and cultural belonging on a series of biological features. Biological features, when apparent, have often caused expulsion, isolation, and stigma. In the past, this has meant that phenotypical features related to a person's physical appearance acquired at birth (like race, or birthplace) or throughout life (a disability, a chronic disease) have served as the basis for establishing attribution. However, the same biological features can establish a membership, or belonging to a community. Historically, a person carrying a disease like leprosy would face removal from the community in which they lived. People affected by the disease would have no other option but to be confined to a remote settlement, where they would form their own—often thriving—communities away from the cities that had expelled them (Frost 2020; Wong 2015). Those affected by HIV/AIDS would face social stigma, as the devastating disease was initially associated with homosexuality and drug use. But the LGBT[2] community built a robust network of solidarity based on the very biosocial qualities that had been used to dismiss and damage it in the first place (Epstein 1996).

[2]While I am aware that this term doesn't reflect today's nomenclature, I am using the historic acronym here.

With the development of genomics and networked societies, the scope of biosociality has expanded to include people with genetic profiles, such as genetic mutations leading to not immediately apparent medical conditions. Thanks to global networks and social media, the possibility of individuals afflicted by the same condition to reach out to each other has increased dramatically. This ability to establish such connections has both produced important networks of solidarity and crucial new research. Individuals sharing the same condition are often very active in raising awareness about their condition, and in doing advocacy and lobbying for increased research funds (Halverson n.d.).

For Wald "the circulation of microbes materializes the transmission of idea. The interactions that make us sick also constitute us as a community" (Wald 2008, 2). Pandemics and infectious diseases may indeed facilitate "the certain formation of new group and individual identities and practices arising out of these new truths" (Rabinow 2008, 183). These can be found in the form of solidarity among equally affected individuals. During the SARS-CoV-2 pandemic, immunocompromised and disabled individuals have become quite vocal about the double threats they had to face: the possibility of contracting COVID-19 could have devastating effects on their health; and the increasing scarcity of medical supplies and hospital beds, and the implementation of a triage-based policy would have endangered their lives ("Disability Visibility Project" n.d.). Similarly, as individuals affected by "long COVID" noticed that their symptoms were dismissed by a medical community too preoccupied with acute care, they formed alliances, exchanged remedies, and sought medical attention and research trials that would ease their discomfort (Barber 2020; Yong 2020a).

As outbreak narratives circulate through refrains and recurring tropes, thus unifying the population under one threat, biosociality empowers differently affected individuals to create advocacy and support groups. But here lies a paradox: The advent of a common threat exhorts collective responses in solidarity with fellow citizens or as part of civic responsibility. Preferred reactions are channeled into top-down recommendations stipulated by medical officers and governments to encourage the population to follow general guidelines, hence protecting themselves and each other. In doing so, these actions prioritize the preferences and desires of a hegemonic homogeneously perceived population, leaving behind many groups, whose experiences are made worse by preexisting conditions and trauma; and dismissing communities for whom pandemics and their symbols acquire a different significance.

Situated Data for Diverse Communities

According to D'Ignazio and Klein, any professional activity implying the management and display of data should consider the situated nature of knowledge and should be able to bring together and embrace multiple or partial perspectives and positionalities to rebalance the hierarchy of "reason over emotion" in data visualization. Widely disseminated and popular maps and graphs tend to contain the view of dominant groups, making assumptions about the behavior and the reactions of entire cities or entire countries. However, pandemics and outbreaks elicit different reactions in different people, have different significance for different communities, and produce painful memories in some individuals or complete dismissal in others.

Looking attentively at the variety of reactions and at the alternative narratives emerging during an outbreak or a pandemic offers a much more comprehensive view of the phenomenon, illuminating non-mainstream stories, and stories reflecting experiences that have been completely forgotten or dismissed. Thus, the re-discovery and re-evaluation of these narratives reveal how inequalities persist even when they are hidden by unified narratives. The recent project *Visualizing the Virus* created by Sria Chatterjee does that by "connect[ing] insights from different disciplines to create a collective digital space" (Chatterjee 2020a). The result is a rich archive of thematically connected spaces where SARS-CoV-2 is seen through a variety of lenses, from visualization to creative imaging, from origin story to conspiracy theories. Besides its interdisciplinary nature, the project is valuable for its ability to map those power dynamics, inequalities (xenophobia, poverty, gender inequalities, lack of healthcare, vaccine imperialism, etc.), and non-hegemonic stories that "viruses make visible."

Visualizing the Virus (Figure 20) to a certain extent is an interdisciplinary epidemiological map, showing the impact of the virus on a population that is not only highly diversified, but also materially, culturally, socially heterogeneous. The project is organized by themed clusters (by general topic, such as art, data visualization, scientific visualization, care, etc.), and curated clusters (clusters grouped by overarching topics aimed to show the inequalities and the ideologies that the pandemic has made visible), where readers can read writing about the origin of the virus and articles on labor under COVID-19; they can view David Goodsell's molecular model of SARS-CoV-2 side by side the seven-frame scroll of Indian painter Swarna Chitrakar, who traveled from village to village to perform stories about an anthropomorphized-looking virus (Chatterjee 2020b).

In *Visualizing the Virus*, continuities and the dispersion of unities resonate together by giving voice to a polyvocal symphony of images and objects, and by opening the space to collective and peculiar narratives, personal and intimate stories. It is to give a voice to personal and diverse stories that British-based artist Anna Dumitriu created *Lockdown Votives,* an installation exploring the impact of the coronavirus on people's lives. For many years, Dumitriu has been studying the history of disastrous pandemics such as the plague, and of devastating infectious diseases such as tuberculosis. While the size and morphology, the treatment and complications of bacteria are very different from the one manifested by

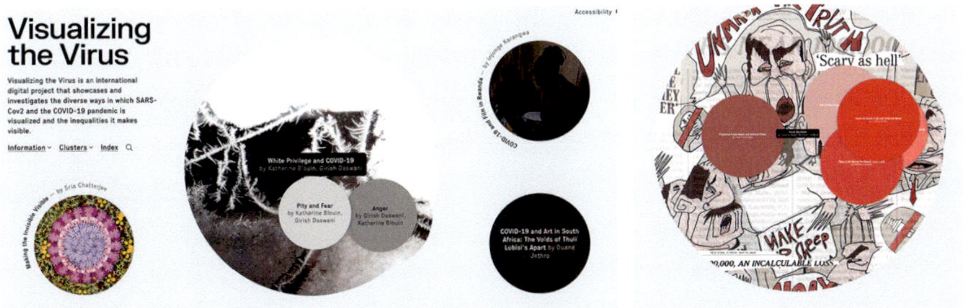

FIGURE 20 *Sria Chatterjee,* Visualizing the Virus, *an international project founded by Dr. Sria Chatterjee. Two screenshots of the website. © www.visualizingthevirus.com.*

viruses, the epidemiological history of viral and bacterial infections share many points in common.

With the spread of SARS-CoV-2, Dumitriu reflected on the way the virus affected people directly or indirectly: the condition of isolation suffered by people suddenly separated from family and friends, the physical vulnerability of immunocompromised individuals, the sudden danger that lockdown would represent for those in abusive relationships, and the long-term effects that some individuals seemed to experience upon contracting the disease. Thus, she resumed and upgraded the series *Ex Voto*, a sort of secular version of votive offerings referencing the religious plaques and paintings created by devotees to give thanks for the fulfillment of a wish (usually the recovery from a disease). In this version, Dumitriu sought stories from friends and colleagues about " … treatment, recovery, and other remembrances" as they related to the first spring 2020 lockdown ("Ex Voto" n.d.). In the installation, engraved votive offerings are hung on a turmeric dyed ribbon which has been a popular remedy during the early stage of the pandemic. The ribbon is impregnated with actual SARS-CoV-2 RNA from a plasmid construct, which the artist obtained from the National Institute for Biological Standards and Control, UK, thanks to a collaboration with researchers Dr. Ines Moura and Dr. Jane Freeman at the University of Leeds who are working with the SARS-CoV-2 primers (ibid.).

Among the votives are vignettes containing the symbols that have characterized the first year of the pandemic: images of hygiene theatre such as sanitizing groceries, images of diseased and infected lungs, oxygen tanks, the elderly. These are all symbols that resonate profoundly and personally with those individuals most affected by the virus and its socioeconomic impact. At the same time, it could mean nothing for other individuals. *Ex Voto* (Figure 21) narrates the stories that cannot make it into a map or a model, or that have been dismissed because they are considered mere anomalies that have nonetheless affected and changed forever the lives of those who have experienced them.

With her work, Dumitriu is interested in narrating stories that can be only partially communicated through maps and models. In the installation *Shieldings* (Figure 22), she reflects on the sharp rise of domestic violence during the coronavirus pandemic. While data clearly reported a staggering 30 percent increase in domestic violence since the start of lockdown in March 2020 (Taub 2020), they were not necessarily given the needed relevance and did not communicate the suffering of many women and other individuals now trapped at home with their abusive partners and family members.

As the artist explains, staying at home placed these individuals in a paradoxical situation: now protected from the virus, they had become vulnerable to another very dangerous threat. Her installation at the old Regent House in Brighton (UK) consisted of thirty miniature beds modeled after the makeshift beds used in the temporary hospitals in Wuhan. Their bedding is hand-dyed using turmeric and walnut husk, the latter a historically popular natural remedy used against the plague. The embroidery, in addition to being a reference to women's traditional domestic activity, represents numbers and "allusions to the idea of data" (Brighton Fringe Festival 2020). Both the location—a house in a clear state of decay—and the reference to the temporary hospitals are reminders of the situation of precarity that these individuals had to face during lockdown.

In an interview with Aristea Fotopoulou, she discusses the important ability of the artist to breath a new life into statistical data through

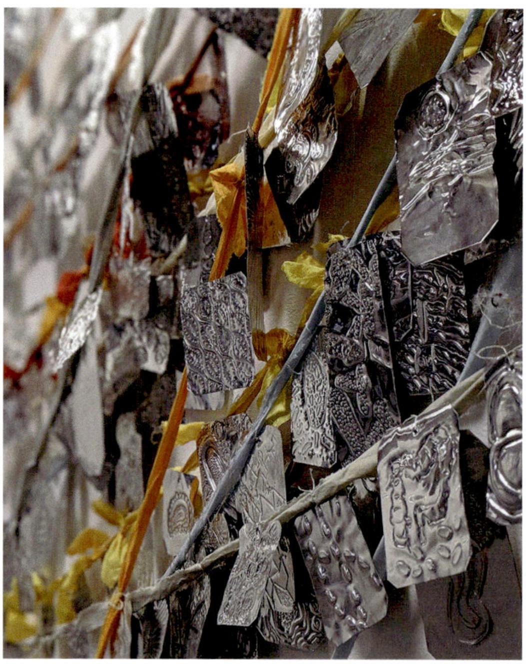

FIGURE 21 *Anna Dumitriu,* Ex Voto, *2020. Detail.* © *Anna Dumitriu.*

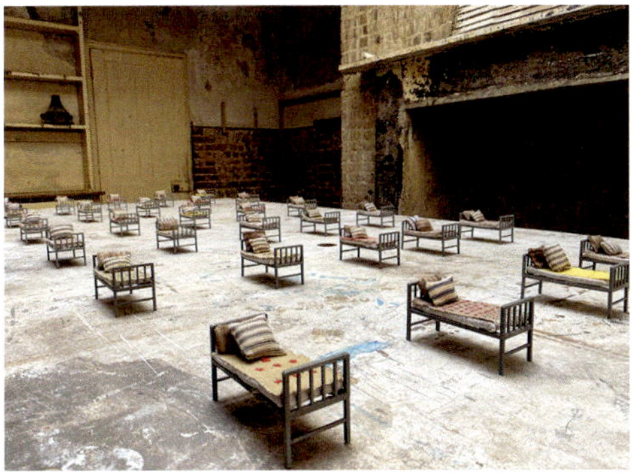

FIGURE 22 *Anna Dumitriu,* Shieldings, *2020. Regent House, Brighton, Brighton Film Festival. © Anna Dumitriu.*

storytelling: ".. people cannot necessarily hold all those figures and those nuances of data in their minds. From the perspective of communicating those data to wider audiences, having a dialogue, and the storytelling, and a narrative is very important. That is something that art can bring to it" (Brighton Fringe Festival 2020). Dumitriu's display gives epidemiological data a physical, three-dimensional appearance, powerfully giving visibility to the story of a group of individuals, whose experiences are too often relegated to mere numbers and statistics. Thus, the installation initiates a dialogue with the audience that would likely not occur, should these data only be presented through traditional data visualization.

In 2019, I attended the show *Public Notice* at the art gallery of Oshawa, curated by Sonya Jones. Inspired by the public notice posters posted on buildings to warn about the "Spanish Flu" in 1818, the exhibition focused on the work of artists who had experienced disease and illness from different perspectives. Ruth Cuthand's series *Trading and Surviving* (Figure 23) was one of them. Her panels featured giant viruses depicted using traditional beadwork. When European settlers established themselves in the Americas, they brought inexpensive beads which they traded in exchange for fur. This uneven exchange also brought infectious diseases such as influenza, measles, smallpox, and other deadly viruses and bacteria. *Trading* examines both sides of European trade. Trade facilitated exchanges between the indigenous populations and British settlers, marking profound transformations in the life and traditions of both. Trade brought new items that transformed and sometimes improved the lives of indigenous populations (Cuthand mentions the iron pot which made boiling food easier to digest, new trapping methods and the horse as a working animal). However, it also caused the decimation of many tribes through disease.

Cuthand's images of viruses and bacteria look familiar, evoking the very outbreak narratives described by Wald. But here, the viruses are not just medical threats and are not limited to infectious diseases. Rather, they reference the viral-like expansion of Colonial British-Canada and their unfair and dishonest trading, as well as the diffuse emotional, physical, and

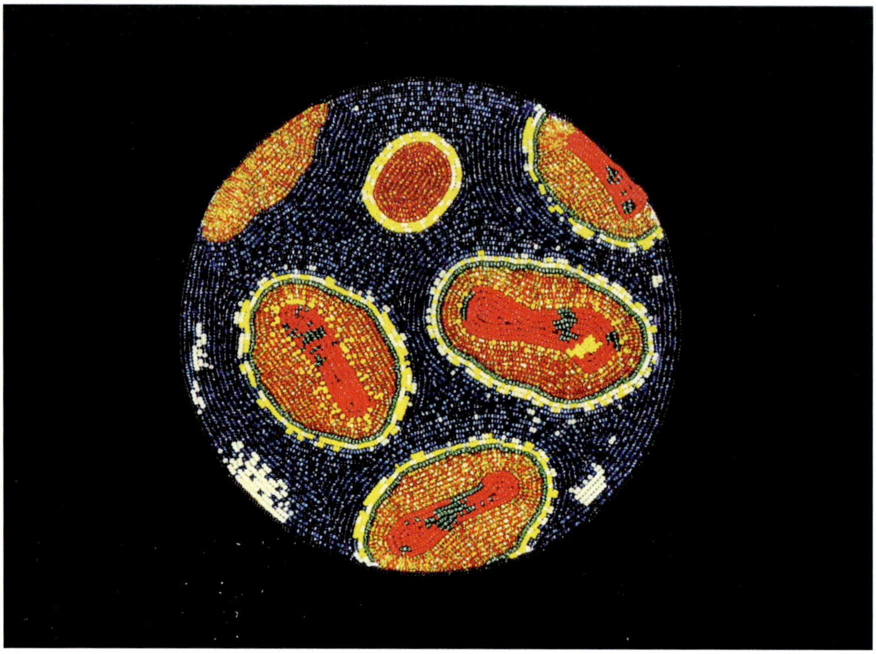

FIGURE 23 *Ruth Cuthand.* SmallPox *from the series* Trading, *2019. Beads and Acrylic on Suedeboard 61.0 × 45.7 cm. Collection of the Mackenzie Art Gallery. © Ruth Cuthand.*

material impact that this expansion brought to the indigenous population. The virus here comes to inhabit the memories and symbols of Cuthand's ancestors.

Similarly to Dumitriu, Cuthand amplifies the stories of a population often marginally represented in official narratives, despite the dramatic effect that infectious diseases had on it. The artist brings these stories to the fore and narrates the multiple meanings that viral phenomena carried for the indigenous population of Canada. Her artwork is a situated epidemiological document. In fact, although it doesn't contain any numbers or statistics, evidence or specimen, it nonetheless is a reminder of the significant role of neglected stories, and the need to move beyond statistics and generalized data to recover the voices of those who have been forgotten.

6

Affective Epidemiologies

During a 2014 episode of WNYC's *On the Media*, host Brooke Gladstone described the similarity between the Ebola outbreak and the pandemics unfolding in movies such as *Oubreak* (1995) and *Contagion* (2011) as uncanny: "As we watch the struggle to contain the Ebola epidemic in West Africa, the images from Liberia, Guinea, and Sierra Leone look hauntingly familiar. Because they are" (*Viral Narratives* 2014). The same images have recurred as Ebola has continued to emerge cyclically in different parts of the African Continent (WHO 2021). Later on, as SARS-CoV-2 unfolded to become a pandemic, similar imagery played before people's eyes worldwide. The following were all recurring items, establishing disturbing parallels between the different pandemics: the view of people wearing hazmat suits (a modern version of the seventeenth-century plague doctor uniform) and health personnel hurriedly performing emergency operations, images of objects such as masks and syringes, colorful molecular models of viruses, and photos of animals and insects as carriers. Metaphors of war and a vocabulary evoking invasion, pemetration, and ongoing battle were regularly used to describe the spread and the effects of outbreaks.

Contagion, a movie released in 2011 and openly inspired by the SARS pandemic of 2001–03, displayed all the above tropes and imagery to provide an accurate, if terrifying, account of how contagion occurs (Jabr 2020). Director Steven Soderbergh had approached epidemiologist Lawrence "Larry" Brilliant to act as a consultant. In March 2020, during the first COVID-19 pandemic wave, the movie rose to the top of the iTunes movies chart (Morris 2020). The images, the symbols, and the behaviors displayed in the news and in the movie—as well as the way they resonated with each other so uncannily—are not new. They are part of a very old reservoir, which is resurrected—updated and adapted—every time an infectious disease emerges to threaten the population, triggering a series of reactions. The same language is also used to describe occurrences that are not necessarily linked to pandemics but similarly affect a large population and spread like one: the rising numbers of people affected by diabetes, obesity, the opioid crisis, and the gun violence epidemic. The same metaphors are repurposed to announce the spread of computer virus and other threats circulating via digital networks.

The use of the same evocative language and the recurring objects and images connect all viral episodes together, fostering a sense of anticipation based on past events and experiences, collective and personal reactions. As Brian Massumi observes, viral phenomena are both virtual and potential: even when the episodes they introduce haven't occurred yet, and sometimes they might not even occur (or partially occur), the symbols they carry may still trigger strong emotional responses (Massumi 2002). Zygmunt Bauman called the reactions inherited from previously occurred or previously narrated outbreaks "recycled fear," exactly because the tropes that accompany viral episodes yet to occur tend to be associated with a collective memory of them, rather than with their real experience (Bauman 2006). At the same time, the images and metaphors accompanying viral episodes are also communicative. They "stick," they sound and feel incisive, they are instinctively and culturally resonant, circulating easily for reasons that sometimes are not entirely clear (Munster 2013). "Refrains are a worlding," Kathleen Stewart (2010) asserts to describe the intensity and density of events, relations, and impacts that repeat and accumulate, showing impressive "capacities to affect and get affected" (339).

In the previous chapter, I described how epidemiology monitors and attempts to predict the spread of infectious diseases and cyberthreats by creating models that use categories and parameters that generalize individuals' behaviors. Models measure the behavior of a homogeneous population, delineating patterns of infections that do not account for exceptional behavior or special cases, thus resulting in the dissemination of projections, not exact predictions. Similarly, the outbreak narratives described by Wald consist of narratives where the use of repetitions and recurring formulas borrowed or inherited from previous pandemics and epidemics unify the message across a population. Epidemiological maps and models contribute to outbreak narratives by creating stories about an impending—medical or networked—threat or by guiding government decision-making and policy changes. I argued that these narratives, as helpful and as compelling as they are, often dismiss the impact of infectious diseases on non-hegemonic groups and their histories, and I called for a more situated kind of epidemiological work that enabled this portion of the population not only to be better represented, but also to be heard.

In this chapter, I move my attention to examining how outbreak narratives mobilize different degrees of affect. The symbols and objects, metaphors and tropes, the refrains and the sound bites used in the perpetuation of outbreak narratives produce very different responses: these may depend on personal and collective experiences of a disease; they may display a range of emotions from fear to anxiety to a sense of inevitability; they may cause individuals to freeze or to dare venturing into the unknown.

To a certain extent, the way that Ruth Cuthand reproduced the evocative images of popular viruses using a traditional beading technique helped her establish a connection between the perceived violence of viral phenomena evoked by the familiar images and the brutal history of colonialism disguised as trade conjured up by the beads. In this chapter, Elaine Whittaker's installations explore how different affective responses emerge from objects and symbols of infectious disease in both scientific accounts and popular culture/cinematic narratives. The narratives simultaneously materialize as collective historical experiences overlapped with personal stories. The series of science fiction performances by Micha Cárdenas and Elle Mehrmand, *Virus.Circus* re-imagine the collective and personal perceptions of viral occurrences, through the choices that people make in the face of the risks viruses pose, treating them as opportunities for dialogue and for creative disruption rather than just as insurmountable and paralyzing obstacles.

Viral Narratives: Metaphors, Objects, and Carriers

Priscilla Wald observes how outbreak narratives have become particularly widespread at the end of the 1980s, with the rise of HIV/AIDS (*Viral Narratives* 2014). The sudden appearance of this new, resilient, and devastating disease effectively eroded the confidence of modern medicine in its ability to annihilate all diseases. From being triumphant and optimistic, the attitude of health professionals and scientists engaged in the fight against infectious diseases seemed to have suddenly come to a halt. This, for Wald, assured that narratives with particularly bleak undertones kept resurfacing and circulating across the media.

Outbreak narratives come to life thanks to " … the repetition of particular phrases, images, and story lines" (Wald 2008, 2), often taking the form of war metaphors, or metaphors that associate the virus with a ruthless villain victimizing the population; semi-fictional origin stories and conspiracy theories; recurring objects or animals immediately associated with a disease or contagion, such as migratory birds, the chicken, the pig; the mask, the syringe, the hazard sign. While the circulation of outbreak narratives, especially the more pessimistic, has increased in intensity since the mid-1980s, this phenomenon is certainly not a novelty. The repertoire of stories created to make sense of mysterious illnesses that seem to hit the population in inexplicably cruel ways is rich, as multiple recurring narratives intersect, shaping the way we understand, describe, and create stories about infectious diseases. Outbreak narratives are equally imposed and spontaneously emerging, brought in by economic and policy needs, personal and collective memory, as well as existing oral history and literature.

The very same repertoire has also been adopted to describe other phenomena and events that spread in fast and uncontrollable ways. The idea of a virus causing outbreaks with dangerous effects was extended to discussing the spread of terrorist cells like ISIS, the abovementioned socially entangled occurrences such as the diabetes epidemic, the gun violence epidemic (Thompson 2017), and the opioid addiction epidemic (Webster, Rice, and Sud 2020). During a conference entitled, "Contagion: exploring modern epidemics," held at Harvard's Radcliffe Institute on October 27, 2017, the latter were explicitly compared to infectious disease outbreaks, with an entire section dedicated to addressing the entanglement of the social with the physiological in the study of all epidemic phenomena, and to acknowledging their similar patterns of diffusion.

The HIV crisis influenced the way computer scientists identified and defined computer viruses too. In his pivotal chapter on the 1988 Morris worm and the rise of computer virus popularity, Andrew Ross documented how during the 1980s direct comparisons between computer viruses and sexually transmitted diseases started proliferating among the computing industry: "The epidemiology of biological virus, and especially AIDS research is being closely studied to help implement computer security plans, and, in these circles, the new witty discourse is laced with references to antigens, white blood cells, vaccinations, metabolic free radicals, and the like" (Ross 1991). This comparison became so common that even the president of the Association for Computing Machinery, in an editorial, "urged attention to 'personal systems hygiene'" (ibid.). The parallel between computer viruses and the AIDS crisis is only partially due to their simultaneous spread in the 1980s. It also pertains to the rise of events that inhibited the confidence of the medical sciences in finding a cure for everything, and the realization that malware could pose a serious threat at a time when computers and networks were increasingly popular, and the computer industry was expanding commercially.

Historically, pandemics and outbreaks generate stories that associate the epidemic with images of war, thanks to stories that had interpreted pandemics such as the plague as a biological weapon launched by enemies (Longrigg 1992). According to Longrigg, we owe the early infectious disease narratives to Thucydides, who documented the 431 BCE plague of Athens in his *History of Peloponnesian War*. Lacking any medical knowledge to explain how epidemics work and where they come from, Thucydides described them as incomprehensible diseases—of divine origins—that "poisoned the body" (Thucydides II 1998, 48). While mentions of plague and pandemics can be found in other earlier texts, Longrigg notes that Thucydides was the first to use war metaphors to describe the behaviors of and the attempts to deal with infectious diseases. These descriptions have since been widely adopted by successive authors and have become not only a stylistic and descriptive model, but also a conceptual prototype for more recent writers.

Longrigg elaborates further, by stating that Thucydides's text did not just describe "the effect of the Plague over Athenians, but also the effect of the Greeks over Plague" (Longrigg 1992, 45). In fact, Thucydides's description of the Athenians' reaction to the unknown epidemic supplied valuable rhetorical models to later literature, establishing a connection between disease (infectious and otherwise) and war, and disease AS war. For instance, Lucretius clearly drew from Thucydides's book in Book VI of *De Rerum Natura* (Lucretius 2020). According to Jason Nethercut (2020), Lucretius's plague narrative is one of the most memorable examples of urban catastrophe in the Roman Empire: in fact, it does not merely refer to the advent of a disease. Lucretius's description of this "mortal Miasma" (Lucr. 6.1138) "encourages his reader to see in the Athenian plague a re-minder that all cities and civilizations will be destroyed, as will the entire world" (Nethercut 2020, 117). Virgil, in book III of *Georgics*, utilized the same expressions used to describe human plagues to chronicle epidemics that did not affect human beings, but cattle (27). Later writers like Campanella, then, in his *Bellum contra Morbum* (Rather 1972) revived the early text consolidating the idea of the battle between human beings and infectious disease as a form of war.

Thucydides used military expressions and war metaphors rhetorically. The later popularity and wide acceptance of these expressions demonstrate how effective they are in describing the fear and anxiety, the struggles, and the hardship that populations hit by epidemic, or individuals afflicted by disease must endure. Their long-term use not only suggested how epidemics should be conventionally narrated, but also how they should be lived. The selective way in which descriptive elements have been extracted from early narratives indicates the authors' commitment to perpetuating specific rhetorical elements. For instance, the way the most recent pandemic is described as a war against SARS-CoV-2—with the work of front-line workers often being likened to "going to war," and "being in the trenches"—simultaneously sounds the alarm in a most incisive way, and eventually persuades the population to follow rules and recommendations (Musu 2020; Panzeri, Paola, and Domaneschi 2021; "*Worse than War*"*: Health Workers on a Year of the Pandemic* [2021]).

The use of war-inspired terms usually assumes that a viral threat is an attacker committing an act of aggression against a population mostly conceived as innocent. The view that there exists a culprit single-handedly attacking an innocent victim is simplistic at best: in fact, while viruses spread mostly thanks to human contact, the origins of the infectious diseases they cause are ecologically complex. Similarly, in computing, although it is technically possible to identify the authors of malware, it is only thanks to users' activity that dissemination takes place. Although the existence of a defined culprit and a clear origin is generally disproved, the urge to find an origin story or to find a culprit persists, leading to beliefs about spreaders and super-spreaders, and, eventually, semi-fictional origin stories and conspiracy theories.

The search for the culprit or the spreader is part of a century-old tradition that downloads responsibility onto enemies (as in the plague of Athens) or onto foreigners or travelers. For instance, Alessandro Manzoni's novel *The Betrothed* (*I Promessi Sposi*) describes the 1630s' Plague of Milan where the "untori" were individuals believed to deliberately spread disease using special ointments applied to the entrance of buildings: "The governor had received a dispatch, countersigned by King Philip IV, warning him to be on the lookout for four Frenchmen, suspected of disseminating poisonous and disease-bearing ointments, who had escaped from Madrid" ("'A Simulated Plague' | Alessandro Manzoni" 2020; Manzoni 1972, 101). At the end of the fifteenth century, a new venereal disease made an appearance in Naples. Until 1530, when poet Girolamo Fracastoro named it "syphilis," the disease was already known by over a dozen names, based on the presumed origin and on the nationality of the foreign traveler who had allegedly introduced it. While in Italy the disease was called French disease, in France it was the Neapolitan Disease; if in Poland it was the German disease, in Germany it was the Polish disease (Hussein 2020). This blame game has survived to this day: Frank Ryan and Tom Koch remind us how Africa and Asia have been historically and stereotypically understood as the sources of major epidemics (Ryan 1997). Asia has been labeled as "Ground Zero" of the avian flu pandemic (*Bulletin of the World Health Organization* 2005); both SARS and SARS-CoV-2 pandemics have caused an outbreak of violence and hate directed against Asians around the world, blaming them for the spread of the disease. Donald Trump further fueled xenophobia against the Asian community by referring to the spread of the SARS-CoV-2 virus from mainland China as the "Chinese Flu" (Lu 2021; Reja 2021).

Bold and repeated statements as well as recurring images are very effective instruments in telling stories about infectious diseases. Origin stories and assumptions inherited from past stories and literature about infection are reflected in the images that appear in the mainstream press and that seem to take a life on their own on social media. For instance, images of carriers associated with the plague are presented in the form of a great number of mice and rats, a reminder of the way these carriers would catch a ride on ships. The carrier is often not alone, but presented as a swarm of mosquitoes, a flock of migrating birds, conveying the idea of a sustained and massive invasion from a queer and alien enemy.

Alternatively, when carriers are assumed to come from farmed animals such as pigs and poultry, as it was the case of the most recent H5N1(avian flu) or H1N1 (swine flu), said animals are seen as being crowded in cages. In this case, the blame is clearly on the handler. In fact, the appearance of these animals refers to the source of the spillover as well as to the farming malpractice, greed, and questionable hygiene practices allegedly causing such spillover. The farm animals displayed in these images strengthen assumptions about their abysmal living conditions. The animal handler living in close proximity with and neglecting to care properly for these animals becomes in part responsible for spreading the disease (Wald 2008; White 2012). Images of wet markets in the first months of 2020 contributed to the narrative that the spillover causing COVID-19 was generated by the consumption of wild animals (the consumption of bat soup, or pangolin meat) or by the extreme proximity of many different live wild animals with each other (in narrow cages) and with humans. It is easy, *Scientific American* reporter Paul Shapiro remarks, to become scandalized by the sight of wet markets in China, as the practice is quite foreign to Western cultures. However, similar unsafe practices are common in industrial farms in North America as well. Shapiro wonders "what kinds of pandemics we may be brewing through own risky animal-use practices" (Shapiro 2020).

Although failing to communicate the ecological and commercial complexities leading to a pandemic, these images produce simple narratives, which temporarily provide straightforward origin stories and simultaneously confirm stereotypes about living habits of a faraway, racialized, and easy to blame population. They serve to justify travel bans and border closures to prevent further spread, thus giving a relative sense of protection to populations. At the same time, they encourage suspicion against travelers and immigrants, and revive xenophobic behavior toward racialized citizens and businesses. It is undeniable how on two distinct occasions SARS (during the 2001 SARS-1 and during the recent SARS-CoV-2 pandemic) caused severe episodes of harassment of Asian citizens and Asian businesses outside of Asia, re-igniting the dormant myths of the "Yellow peril" and of the untrustworthy immigrant (Y. Li and Nicholson Jr. 2021; White 2012).

Whether through metaphors, images, and other memorable storylines, outbreak narratives both reflect and suggest how a society lives and perceives the spread of infectious diseases and pandemics. Even in uneventful times or times of relative health, these narratives never completely disappear. In the same way the viral permeates a variety of new phenomena, adding them to its repertoire, it also inherits and appropriates narratives and metaphors from the past to describe them. Neil Gerlach and Sheryl Hamilton observed that more recently the production of these narratives has not only extended beyond medical circumstances but has resulted in an ".. explosion of communication about imagined, potential pandemics." This overproduction, which they call pandemic culture, effectively leads to "an affective state resulting from living in conditions of constant vulnerability to infection, or feeling as though one is" (Gerlach and Hamilton 2014). Christos Lynteris goes even further when he talks about a pandemic imaginary, that is, an imaginary based on a worse-case scenario where increasingly frequent zoonotic infectious diseases may lead to humanity's final demise (Lynteris 2020).

It is true that the exponential increase in narratives referring to social vulnerability caused by potential pandemics and other pandemic-scale cataclysms (what Gerlach and Hamilton call "diseaseability") may influence collective behavior, promoting modes of living dominated by a biopolitical discourse that favors preventative and pre-emptive actions rather than more instinctive or unstructured behavior. However, these narratives are also non-binding and remarkably generative: as Stewart remarks, "modes of attending to scenes and events spawn socialities, identities, dream worlds, bodily states and public feelings of all kinds" (Stewart 2007, 10). The refrains and automatisms that allow these narratives to go viral do not form a unifying discourse but acquire very different meanings to different people and don't always produce the same reactions.

From Outbreak Narratives to Communicable Narratives

When a video or a media product surprisingly gains widespread popularity, we say that it is "going viral," just like a virus does. Anna Munster lists the three aspects characterizing the viral: "speed of spread, quantity of views or users accessing something being spread, and the unpredictability of what will spread" (Munster 2013, 100). If for pioneers like Douglas Rushkoff "going viral involved stickiness and riskiness" (101) that is, it had to contain subversive elements throughout popular culture, for Munster this is not or no longer the case. She observed that a viral event doesn't need to manifest specific characteristics; all it needs to be transmitted widely is a particular type of unquantifiable and unspoken affectivity, a visceral quality, a "condition in which the biological, the communicative and the affective pass between one another" (Munster 117). For Munster, "instances of going viral are moments that have not been deliberately orchestrated by viral marketing campaigns. Instead, they erupt out of nowhere, gather momentum, and behave like the dynamics of nonlinear systems" (117). Communicability, rather than communication, enables their transmission among individuals. Communicability implies the circulation of clues that are detached and deterritorialized from a specific event but resonate at all levels of affective or material information. While these clues don't need scientific data or plausible representations to trigger a reaction, they are often strategically used to reinforce a message: for instance, the red circles chosen by the team who created the Johns Hopkins map were a strategic clue used to make the message of an expanding pandemic more incisive and explicit.

In some way, tropes and metaphors from past pandemics go viral when they lose their specificity and remain in circulation to describe new pandemics and other viral phenomena. Perhaps, it is the very loss of specificity that enables their remarkable adaptation. Individuals may respond to "clues" evoked by popular and collective understandings of certain phenomena. Their responses might also be based on their personal experiences with these phenomena. Clues may be triggered by a familiar symbol, or they may originate from a movie, or a documentary. These clues don't necessarily provide more information about a pandemic but are still able to awaken a reaction in the individual.

Since as early as 2006, multidisciplinary artist Elaine Whittaker has worked with "sites of microbial visitations" (Whittaker n.d.), that is, iconic objects standing in for infection transmission or generally evoking apprehension towards infectious diseases. Whittaker devoted a good part of her artistic career to studying the manifestation and the impact of infectious diseases and outbreaks on society and on individuals. In her 2006 exhibition at the Redhead Gallery in Toronto, a large number of mosquitos (*The Swarm*) (Figure 24) encased in an encaustic *tableau* warned the public of their potential for carrying and transmitting serious diseases; chicken bones (*Zoonosis*) (Figure 25) formed a sculpture to remind us that some of the most devastating influenza pandemics were carried by avian hosts; a nautical vessel (*Microbial Passage*) evoked memories of travel and of the potentially lethal castaways that these ships unknowingly carried; and a large number of protective masks (*Miasma*) indicated the attempt to protect oneself from the spread of infectious diseases. These masks were hand-painted with pictures of the most popular viruses and disease-causing bacteria to indicate that while we try to protect ourselves from specific diseases, numerous more are waiting for us, sometimes residing inside our masks and our bodies.

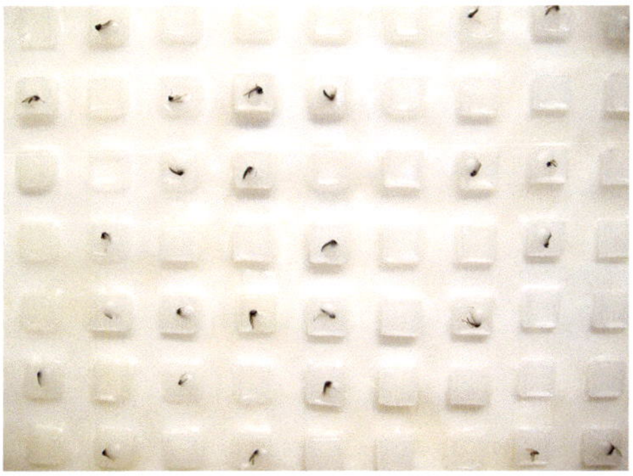

FIGURE 24 *Elaine Whittaker,* The Swarm. *© Elaine Whittaker.*

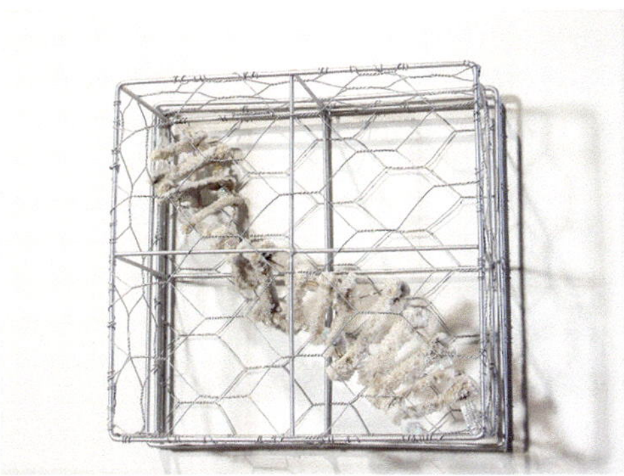

FIGURE 25 *Elaine Whittaker,* Zoonosis, *2006. 68"×10"×5" Chicken wire, chicken bones, beads, and grown salt crystals. © Elaine Whittaker.*

These objects are no simple list of dreadful items. They are the sites of microbial visitations, that is, the interfaces separating and connecting infectious diseases and human hosts. They are the "clues" instantaneously conjuring up ideas of contagion and infectious disease transmission, causing certain visceral reactions or invoking attraction described by Munster. As Whittaker gathered mosquitoes, chicken bones, and other objects, she formed a basic census of elements that usually come to mind when one talks about outbreaks and other infectious episodes. Displayed all together, they did not evoke one unified and universal narrative, but allowed the visitor to make connections based on their own personal experiences and their interpretations of these tropes.

To conjure up connections between objects and narratives, the artist covered part of the collection of items with colonies of *halobacteria*, a type of archaea with an aerobic metabolism requiring a highly concentrated salt environment. She chose this organism for its ability to grow, its resemblance to sea salt, and its connection to travel at sea and explorations. As well, she picked it because of its visual appearance, which gives a sense of creating "infectious-like botches" (Roach Pierson 2007). The omnipresence of *halobacteria*'s growth across Whittaker's installations as a unifying medium reveals three overarching themes cutting across her work. Their presence stands for the dense travel of infectious events among individuals in proximity to each other. It reveals how transmission also occurs figuratively, through iconic objects and collective memories. Finally, it shows how transmission and infection may follow different paths, thus generating different narratives and invoking unique personal stories.

This *halobacterium* can be found in the exhibitions *Dreadful Visitations* (2006), *Spontaneous Generation* (2007), *Ambient Plague* (2013), and *Shiver* (2015). In these exhibitions, each object can be seen as modular, standing for one of the many aspects comprising much more complex narratives. To a certain extent, the objects in Whittaker's exhibitions recall the way that tropes, images, and storylines recur as outbreak narratives. In fact, some of the items from the *Dreadful Visitations* exhibition were exhibited as stand-alone artworks, some were incorporated in audio-video collaborations, or were carried on, expanded, and incorporated into later installations. This is the case of the masks known as *Miasma* (Figure 26): they were originally hanging as a group of objects, carrying colorful gouache micrographs of a variety of lethal and infectious diseases. In "*Shiver*," the artist wears them in a series of photographs titled "*Screened For*" (Figure 27). The series was later assembled (a collaboration with Julia Krolik and Owen Fernley) and exhibited as a one-minute silent film sequence at Toronto Urban Film Festival in 2016. Recently, the work acquired remarkable popularity during the initial phase of the 2020 coronavirus pandemic, appearing on magazine covers and in online exhibitions. The transformation of this work, like that of several other objects appearing in Whittaker's installations, can be compared to the trajectory and transformation of outbreak narratives: they are displayed, then adapted to later circumstances, or incorporated into other installations, adding to, contrasting, interacting with, or complementing newer objects.

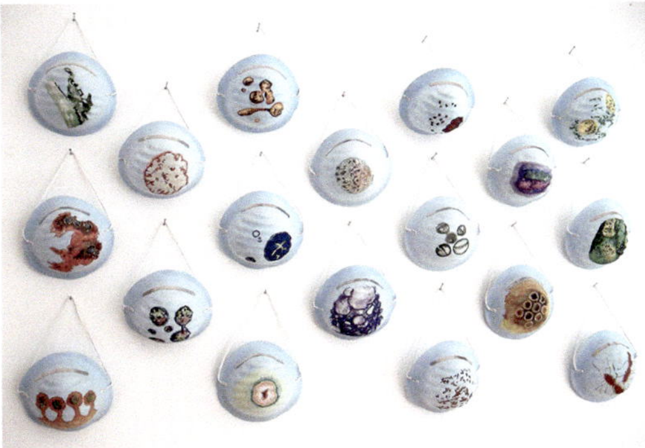

FIGURE 26 *Elaine Whittaker,* Miasma, *2006. Guache and 123 respiratory masks. © Elaine Whittaker.*

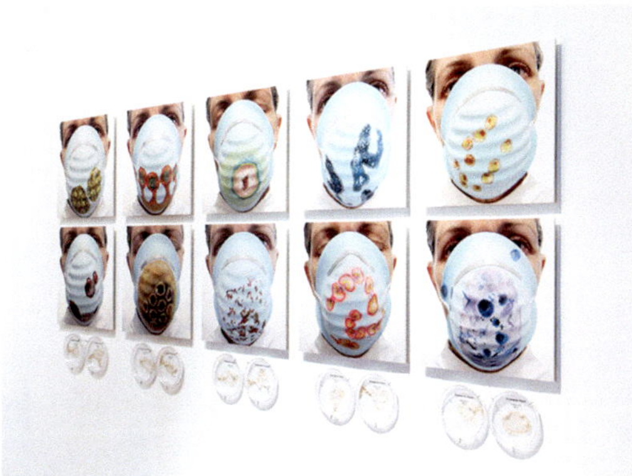

FIGURE 27 *Elaine Whittaker,* Screened For. *Photographic Series. Digital Prints. RedHead Gallery, 2015. © Elaine Whittaker.*

Affect and the Unseen

In September 2013, the RedHead Gallery opened the exhibition *Ambient Plagues*. Visitors were welcomed by a profusion of Petri dishes which occupied two walls at the remotest corner of the gallery. Titled *I Caught It at the Movies* (Figure 28), the Petri dishes display contained stills from well-known movies belonging to the genre of dystopian sci-fi movies that focus on contagion and pandemics. This included *Outbreak, Contagion, The Andromeda Strain, 28 Days Later*, and others. Nearby, the installation displayed other Petri dishes, containing hand-painted reproductions of microphotographs and molecular models of notorious viruses and infectious pathogens (HIV, rabies, flu, etc.).

In Whittaker's installations, Petri dishes, syringes, and other objects that routinely populate the imagination pertaining to infectious diseases are not just isolated refrains, "being of sensation" or a "composition of percepts and affects that catches on" (Munster 2013). They form a kaleidoscopic ecology reflecting both the material and the symbolic spread of infections,

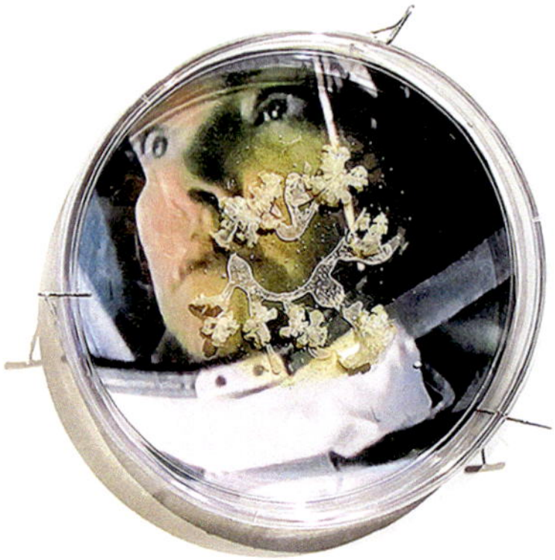

FIGURE 28 *Elaine Whittaker,* I Caught It at the Movies. *Halobacteria on printed Petri dishes. Exhibited respectively at Ambient Plague 2013 and FACTT Toronto 2018. © Elaine Whittaker.*

showing how the same narratives that infiltrate the scientific field, merge with popular culture in often imperceptible and surreptitious ways. In doing so, they expose both collective responses, and more intimate reactions to infectious diseases.

The pairing of such a variety of dissimilar items provided an opportunity for the spectators to contemplate their very own inability to disentangle aesthetic elements and scientific data, technical information and popular culture, the characteristics of individual pathogens and their generalized and vaguely defined pandemic qualities. The disappearing boundaries of, and between, the objects on display, the scientific process, and the cinematic narratives referenced in this exhibition occurred at the physical, disciplinary, and discursive level.

This disintegration not only reveals the extent to which science and fiction share rhetoric and symbols, but also underlines the power of these objects to generate a range of different and often alternating feelings: these Petri dishes could generate curiosity and speculative thoughts about the resemblance between the different clues they represent; they could be the cause of different degrees of anxiety and fear; they could unify the audience through their collective anxieties.

Whittaker's body of work is emblematic of how the responses to infectious phenomena are as much collective as they are individual; they are profoundly diversified and situated. Her series can be interpreted as an object-oriented affective epidemiology. Affect, here starts from what Sara Ahmed (2010) calls the "messiness of the experiential, the unfolding of bodies into worlds, and the drama of contingency, how we are touched by what we are near" (30). Instead of data and viral trajectories, Whittaker displays objects capturing a range of emotions and a variety of visceral and even physical reactions to viral phenomena.

Whittaker injects most of her installations with personal memories and impressions on infectious diseases. This gesture invites, even elicits, the participatory responses of the audience, encouraging them to identify with and recollect the imaginary stories emerging from the objects displayed in the installation. Her work equally emphasizes the collective and diverse nature of lived and subjective viral narratives, promoting them in opposition to the de-personalized and standardized line of action and reaction recommended by institutions and organizations.

This is the case with her 2018 installation *Contained*, where Whittaker grapples with her mother's journey as a patient affected by tuberculosis and her subsequent painful experience in a Quebec sanatorium. *Contained* documents a personal story. At the same time, it is a reflection on the politics of containment and restraint, that is, on the fact that containing a disease or an outbreak means also taking measures that segregate, isolate, exclude, and impart pain upon populations and individuals; it takes into account the different ways in which facing an outbreak will be experienced. In her own words, *Contained* means "holding something or someone in place. Keeping proper control. Limiting expansion. Preventing advancement. When an infectious disease presents itself, we act to contain it. An act that can be both liberating and traumatic" (Whittaker 2018). *Contained* is an installation that encompasses both these possibilities. As well, it illustrates the unfolding of a journey living with and carrying tuberculosis, incorporating historical information about the disease and its treatment, public assumptions and stigma, as well as personal suffering and painful memories associated with it.

Whittaker's installations display what Barbara Maria Stafford once called "the unseen," that is, not only that which escapes—material or metaphorical—visibility, but also that which current language cannot describe or articulate. The unseen is not caused by the absence of adequate technical instrumentation, although the lack of instruments to measure and visualize an epidemic or the structure of a virus goes hand in hand with the unspeakable ephemerality and uncertainty that dominate said virus.

In examining scientific and medical images of the body disseminated in the seventeenth century, Stafford observes how its iconographical tradition (Stafford 1993b) had a keen interest in capturing and transmitting elements such as fear, pain and discomfort, insidious danger and terror. These only to a certain extent constitute subjective or aesthetic interpretations of the effects of a disease on the individual. They are also attempts to record and to map its symptomatic course. Being at that time the only observable evidence available of the passage of a mysterious entity through the human body, these visual accounts retained scientific value to help diagnose and identify current and future similar diseases. Besides their scientific merits, these medical chronicles contained added elements that exceeded the immediate determination of a diagnosis: for example, they did not shy away from reproducing the practitioner's personal interpretation of the suffering of the patient, the distaste for the grotesque manifestations of the disease, and the anxiety regarding a disease that could be potentially dangerous for the clinician and for other individuals. The attention to morbid details and the physical degradation described in these chronicles equally unlocked pity for, or stigmatized, the victims.

The recurring elements in Whittaker's installations, in their different manifestations, reveal different instances of the unseen. The animals and the vessels allegedly carrying mysterious epidemics, the objects (the masks), and the substances (the *halobacteria*) bring to life different ideas of contagion and different degrees of anxiety and fear; they may evoke a sense of disgust or physical discomfort triggered by direct personal and familiar experiences with disease and pandemic.

Borrowed and Anticipated Reactions

The objects and images contained in Whittaker's installations do not address specific viral phenomena but include clues and insights clearly pointing to themes related to contagion. The title of the installation, *I Caught It at the Movies*, suggests various ideas of communicability: what does the viewer catch at the movies? While the short sentence may remind us of the common expression "catching a cold," in the context of this exhibition, it may also evoke other indistinct viral phenomena, such as past pandemics that we haven't experienced, but that have survived in the collective memory for many years, losing their specific meaning, but becoming linked with apparently unrelated events and objects (Bauman 2006; Buiani 2014; Longrigg 1992).

As a matter of fact, many of the recurring viral narratives we find in news media and in some scientific discourse could as well be describing any viral phenomenon that simultaneously has already occurred and hasn't occurred yet. In fact, a great deal of metaphors, storylines, and imagery about viral phenomena derive from early accounts or historical descriptions of epidemics. Epidemiology itself bases a lot of the early information about developing infectious diseases on historical data of past epidemics. The analysis of past events has proved to both provide important information about the forms and the manifestation of epidemics to come, and have helped build early projections about developing pandemics. As observed in Chapter 5, most warnings and alerts one can find on infection maps are partially based on historical data. For instance, early COVID-19 pandemic maps and molecular models of SARS-CoV-2 used data from the 2003 SARS pandemic (GISP and Geraghty 2020; Falconieri Hays 2020).

While certainly useful, the use of past narratives and historical data to anticipate upcoming viral episodes may result in enhanced anxiety. Bauman

(2005) called this a derivative or "second-hand" form of anxiety, a "socially and culturally recycled fear," a " … sediment that outlives the encounter and becomes an important factor in shaping human conduct even if there is no longer a threat to life or integrity … derivative fear acquires a self-propelling capacity" (3). This is especially true when past viral episodes are particularly devastating. For instance, Jessica Otis contends that "Covid-19 is not the plague, but many of our experiences today would have been familiar to anyone who survived one of the plague epidemics that routinely swept through early modern Europe" (Otis 2020). The first event comes to be seen as a sort of blueprint for the second, and so there is a modeling of reactions to the second based on the recollections of the first. In this way, a particular health emergency or viral incident that occurred in the past can trigger reflex reactions, which pre-date and anticipate the existence of current events, fostering various preventive actions.

The memory of the human casualties caused by the infamous 1918 "Spanish" flu has become the precedent used to justify predictions about possible future outbreaks. The 1918 Spanish flu decimated over 25 million people (although statistics vary) (WHO, n.d.). There has been a great deal of study of the virus that caused the flu, of the effects of the disease, and how it spread. A 2005 WHO bulletin confirmed that although flu pandemics are substantially unpredictable, epidemiological analysis showed that pandemic incidents are usually cyclical. Gupta predicted that "in the next 20 year or 30 years there will be a pandemic and it will have the potential to bring humanity to its knees" (Gupta 2017). Every year, flu season came with scientists wondering if when the "big one" would unfold. Despite the expectations, it would have been nearly impossible to predict the current pandemic.

There is no reliable way to establish with certitude the future course of the most recent flu strains, Kamps and Reyes-Terán, admitted, echoing both WHO and CDC:

> As unpredictable as influenza pandemics are, as unpredictable is the virus itself. We know nothing about the pathogenic potential of the next pandemic strain. The next pandemic may be relatively benign, as it was in 1968 and 1957, or truly malignant, as was the 1918 episode. We don't know if the next pandemic will be caused by the current bête noire, H5N1, or by another influenza strain. We ignore how the next pandemic will evolve over time, how rapidly it will spread around the world, and in how many waves. We don't know which age groups are at the highest risk of severe outcomes. We have no idea whether the next pandemic will kill 2, 20, or 200 million people.
>
> (Kamps and Reyes-Terán 2006)

The worry about the possible worldwide spread of the H5N1 avian flu (which, the WHO assured, "does not jump easily from birds to humans or spread readily and sustainably among humans" [WHO, n.d.]) was driven, in part, by its similarities with the Spanish flu strain: both were identified as zoonotic viruses, sharing the same avian origins (Crawford 2000; Goudsmit 2004; WHO n.d.). It is no surprise that the spread of the COVID-19 global pandemic has been accompanied by continuous references to the 1918 flu.

Although no event can happen with identical modalities, a few salient elements are sufficient to prompt the recognition of a certain type of phenomenon, and to elicit a reaction that will lead to the implementation of certain prophylactic measures. The "trigger moment" is what Massumi calls a re-presentation of an emotion, that is, an "anticipatory repetition of an affective event, precipitated by the encounter between the body's irritability and a sign" (Massumi 2005, 40).

Threats, Massumi reminds us, are "cultivated," acquiring real status not through effective occurrence, but through anticipation (Massumi 2002). Even though these phenomena exist only in a virtual form, they have the ability to cause great anxiety. In fact, they are also "potential" (Massumi 2002). Their virtual quality can be perceived as very real, for it can refer to an abstract, yet to be formally acknowledged, object. The potential in viruses is therefore in a constant state of becoming—it might not even occur (58). Infections are monitored with apprehension, not because of the effective danger they represent, but because of the anticipation of the disastrous effects they could have. The case of the mathematical models I examined in the previous chapter is a case in point: starting from real or historical data, they create projections based on potentials. As soon as a risk becomes a reality, it ceases to be simply a risk.

Fear generated by past events and further predictions is then a reaction to a "quasi-cause" (Massumi 2005, 35) that hasn't manifested yet. It is the product not of something that already exists as "Potential is unprescripted. It only feeds forward the registering of an event" (Massumi 2002, 9). Potential is "one with becoming," as opposed to the possibility of the event, which constitutes its coming into shape, its manifestation (Massumi 2005, 10–11). Sooner or later (or never), in a time and space that is unknowable and impossible to predict (although hypotheses and predictions are countless), viruses, in the form of an emerging infectious disease, or as powerful and skillfully designed computer worms, or as a brilliantly designed ad campaign, will likely (or not) strike, with consequences that may (or may not) be disastrous. Even when the potential for their realization is remote, it is looming.

The ambiguity that characterizes the reporting of and warnings about past and potential pandemics is the product of many intersecting biopolitical vectors: it is in part the design of local and international public health agencies and governments to make a convincing argument that will compel the population to make unanimous choices. The population may or may not choose to follow directions and recommendations. Importantly, most recommendations become law in case of emergencies, with a few exceptions: travel advisories tend to be applied unevenly and arbitrarily and have become bans only for those traveling from countries deemed dangerous because they have been affected by a pandemic. One may recall, for example, the responses from Citizen and Immigration Canada to immigrant agricultural workers coming from the H5N1 (swine flu) pandemic "ground zero": in this case, containing the virus by temporarily preventing these workers from entering Canada or by quarantining them was deemed unnecessary as it would be damaging to regional and transnational trades and the national businesses in need of this labor force. Melissa Autumn White defined this decision paradoxical, because it was dictated by economics and not by medical concern (White 2012).

The arrangement of contradictory statements converging in the viral discourse is also a manifestation of real concerns caused by the material difficulties in predicting the outcome of outbreaks and the failure to provide definite information about viruses' spread. These remain important factors generating greater amounts of anxiety as well as suspicion and distrust of science and the authorities. Recommendations often tend to dispense vague and general suggestions (wash your hands, wear a mask, be mindful of your surroundings). This tentativeness has contributed in maintaining, not easing the continuous sense of anxiety accompanying epidemic events and a generalized suspicion of any source of information that claims to advise on the topic of infectious diseases. These suggestions coming from public health are also undermined by transforming science, and by new findings that might literally undermine or even contradict what we knew before. These developing situations may require changes in policy, or even suggest opposite recommendations. A case in point is the debate on whether SARS-CoV-2 is airborne, resulting in ambiguous statements about the effectiveness of masks, and later in adverse reactions to the changing rules obliging the population to wear them in public (Khazan 2021; J. R. Raymond 2020).

Conflicting statements create inconsistencies within a given discourse, by referring to different authorities, and different regimes of truth. In the resulting amalgamation of different statements and expressions of different forces (power-relations), power is "never in anybody's hands" (Deleuze 2006, 89), as all forces "are always in the position of undergoing and exercising this power" (99) in a rather concerted way. This understanding of power is also the manifestation of affect, "since force defines itself by its very power to affect other forces to which it is related, and to be affected by other forces" (71). Since power "passes through the hands of the mastered no less than through the hands of the masters (since it passes through the hands of every related force)" (72), it must manifest through a principle of cohesion. Disseminating conflicting statements becomes therefore a principle of cohesion in itself that "organizes the discourse and restores to it its hidden unity" (Foucault 1989a, 167). Viral phenomena, in their material and metaphorical provisional nature, remain caught in an eternal loop.

It is not possible to differentiate between attempts to understand and cope with viruses and attempts to manipulate their reception to obtain economic and political advantages, between elements suggesting real anxiety and concerns about the spread of viruses, and elements aiming at opportunistically reproducing such fear. In fact, to argue that the idea that the perpetuation of indeterminacy and provisionality in epidemiological maps and visual accounts is the product of calculated manipulation is to dismiss the very definition of fear and how fear affects not only the receiver of these accounts but also those who fabricate them and disseminate them. The modulation of fear can be both inadvertent and purposeful. Experts, after all, are aware that the information they are about to disseminate is subject to various margins of error; they are aware that information is not 100 percent accurate.

The apparent reliability of the data collected to track viruses and of the maps generated from that data is undermined by their ultimate fallibility, because determining the future trajectory of viruses is dependent on too many factors. Should the public blindly trust those who claim that the latest flu X will be the next human pandemic? Should they trust warnings about the dangers of a faraway pandemic, or the latest news about a circulating computer threat, or the latest recommendations regarding preemptive actions or protection protocol? For every reassuring sentence that downplays the dangerous potential of viruses, there are corresponding statements that undermine or contradict it. As a result, we are left with an unclear idea of what viruses and their effects are.

Affect, Anticipation, Rebellion

Set in an imaginary dystopian future dominated by fear of contagion and where infections are considered a crime to be punished with quarantine and prison time, Micha Cárdenas and Elle Mehrmand's series of performances (titled *Virus.Circus.Breath; Virus.Circus.Touch; Virus.Circus.Meme*) are prophetic and visionary at the same time. The two artists walk us into a laboratory. As they enter, we learn that they are living in a sanitized society paralyzed by a fear of potential infections. Even the common cold is considered a threat. One of the protagonists recalls having "witnessed combots transfer civils suspicious of being infected to the federal penitentiary ... some are infected with the rhinovirus, which used to be known as the common cold" (Cárdenas 2011, 111). The protagonists, too, fall victim to this anxiety, as there is no immediate way of knowing if their daring behavior will cause any contagion. Acknowledging the risks that such activity will entail, they pay attention to any small change, as any detail can make a difference: "Aware again of your physical safety, you see a bit of glass on your latex glove and step back quickly, shaking it off. Your breath is hot and smelly now; the fear mobilizing compounds in your saliva, thanks to inherited evolutionary mechanisms" (113).

Once in the lab, using found objects and monitoring systems creatively, the two protagonists learn how to engage in erotic experiments without skin-to-skin contact (Cárdenas 2011). Touching and sexual intimacy are the most extreme and dangerous behaviors one can entertain in case of an outbreak. This situation creates a tension between the apprehension of becoming ill from the exchange of sex toys and human fluids and the desire to explore "bodily autonomy, despite narratives of power that seek to determine a person's corporeal experience before one has had a chance to define the body oneself" (Cárdenas 2011, 54).

The audience, too, participates in this scene. Following an introduction during which the audience is warned to wear a mask against possible contagion, *Virus.Circus* unfolds a narrative that is only partially unfamiliar to its public. While the scene takes place in a futuristic setting of mixed reality dense with technological devices (as the live action is matched with Second Life[1] simultaneous interaction between the protagonists' avatars), and attempts at "reconfiguring their notions of intimacy" (55), the issues it raises are definitely contemporary. As Kroker (2006) suggests, we are already living in a world where these measures are not-too-subtly being implemented: for instance, the "trusted traveler" program at American airports, the immunization of the body politic against the threat of domestic and foreign terrorism, and the protection of the "American homeland" from the threat of viral contagion, are all products of viral narratives as much as they are of military narratives. Thus, the rhetoric of war, the discourse on terrorism, and viral narratives merge to become a "convenient *tromp-d'oeil* for the advent of the biometric state," where citizens are willing to give away all their freedom for the sake of safety and security. These are all narratives that have sadly become very familiar during the recent COVID-19 pandemic, as the metaphor of war—a metaphor very dear to the medical field—has become a favorite in describing the difficulties and the challenges that the virus has caused to people and the economy. Similarly, the need to contain the spread of the disease produced debates on the choices and the risks that contact tracing and surveillance would pose to civil liberties.

In their use of science fiction and virtual worlds (Second Life), Mehrmand and Cárdenas's work was inspired from Blast Theory's alternate reality as code switching between mixed and alternate reality. Their goal was to "draw you into a terrain where slightly different codes might be at work" creating "a new world but at the same time enable[ing] you to see the real world through a new lens" (Cárdenas 2011, 32; Juliano 2010). This strategy, in a way, is reminiscent of the strategies of "deterritorialization" and "subjectivation" once described by Felix Guattari. In *Chaosmosis,* Guattari draws inspiration on his experience working at the La Borde Clinic, where the psychotic patients were encouraged to practice activities with which they were completely unfamiliar. According to Guattari, this type of

[1]An online multimedia platform founded in 1999 that allows the user to create an avatar to interact with other users. Although its popularity has waned in the past ten years, as of 2023, the virtual world is still populated by over 60 million active users.

activity became a "production *sui generis*" (Guattari 1995, 6) because the patients confronted "a new material of expression," and the "constitution of complexes of 'subjectivation': multiple exchanges between individual, group, machine." Offering the patient a way out of their repetitive patterns, this strategy proposed a "new aesthetic paradigm" that would allow them "new modalities of subjectivity in the same way an artist creates new forms from the palette." For Guattari, this opportunity represented a process that led to the realization of "autonomy or *autopoiesis*" (7) of the patient. This mechanism of re-territorialization and re-location not only provides many insights into the processes that enable the formation and transformation of subjectivity, but also its potential to move away from the constraints of fixed mechanisms and patterns.

Guattari calls these mechanisms hegemonic "collective territorialized subjectivity" (Guattari 1995, 34) that attracts, encircles, and crystallizes one object into a particular limited space by folding "one universe of value into another in a general movement of folding over on itself" (102). By doing this, a particular type of discourse becomes institutionalized as a "territorialized assemblage of enunciation" (98). For instance, the alterity and negativity of viruses, along with the generalized anxiety they produce, lead to the maintenance of an epistemological, ontological, and political status quo.

In their performances, Mahrmand and Cárdenas inserted viral narratives of fear into a *transreal* setting, that is, into a scenery that is both fictional and sensational, as well as non-fictional (in this case, a fictional background and story with a non-fictional set of themes). Their goal was to draw attention to the narratives of power that occur in these circumstances. Also, they aimed to "present audiences with acts and scenarios that are unfamiliar to them, reconfiguring their notions of intimacy to include detailed biometric readouts and pixelated body avatar bodies, deterritorializing their ideas of sex in which the amorous partners never touch each other or only touch each other with metal instruments" (Cárdenas 2011, 55).

While official and mainstream accounts tend to conceal—hardly and awkwardly—affective elements behind the authoritative voice of institutionalized knowledge, in their works, Whittaker, on the one hand, and Cárdenas & Mehrmand, on the other, don't shy away from making them explicit. In both cases, personal experience, the sense of indeterminacy caused by the volatile nature and spread of viruses, and a drive toward rebelling against it are emphasized as crucial aspects of the artwork.

In Cárdenas & Mehrmand's work, the protagonists stage their hesitation between finally engaging in intimate physical relations using the tools found in the dusty lab, and the fear that one of those tools will make them sick. This aspect raises issues of trust and reminds us of the many variables, the anticipation, and the layers of indeterminacy that characterize the invisible presence of viruses and the mechanism of spread of epidemics.

The two characters in *Virus.Circus* choose to rebel. It is not the viral threat that disturbs the two protagonists, but the very ban on physical contact and the fact that this prevents them from engaging in any intimate encounter. In reflecting on the frustration and desire of the protagonist, one can't help but thinking of the longing for human contact, and for each other that people experienced during lockdown in the spring 2020. Even those aware of the risk they would take by engaging in closer, non-social distanced, intimate relationships were left with an urge to reconnect and to find strategies for re-establishing contact. During the performance, it is exactly this unease, and the protagonists' burning desire that led them to overcome the barriers erected by imposed rules of conduct and behavioral constraints.

After having evoked the scene of people being imprisoned because of being infected with the rhinovirus, one of the characters asks: "If it was so common, how bad could it be?" (111). This is an invitation for transgression and a plea to repeat the transgression. When in doubt about whether to use the tools (and thus take a risk), and/or do nothing (thus walking away), they choose the first option, a disregard for the rules that pay back in the form of new experiences and pleasure.

"Amidst the collapse of information capitalism, before the myth of rigid national borders was finally eradicated in an instant by the N3N91 mutations ... they experimented with their bodies, applying Do-it-yourself and Do-it-together ethos to medical science to imagine what might lie beyond all they knew" (110).

Reversed Narratives

Whittaker's infectious series and *Virus.Circus* contain all the stereotypical elements that invoke infectious diseases and that persist today to different degrees in different forms of visual and literary expressions. Neither work contains any geographical or territorial references, data, or specific references, as if they were suspended in space. The contagion acquires a universal significance. But it is because of this very aspect that the spectators can let their imagination run wild.

What if the outbreak narratives, the collectivization of fear, the surveillance of self and other were turned upside down? What if they encouraged us to excavate and speak about personal stories, fears, and even hopes, instead of a de-personalized group? Elle Mehrmand and Micha Cárdenas's daring series *Virus.Circus*, and of Elaine Whittaker's "contagious" cycle, are impressive examples of how outbreak narratives in the form of both collective and personal responses to pandemics have been incorporated into artistic practices, and how "the cultural and social ecologies" (Whittaker n.d.) of epidemics and infectious diseases affect us often in uncontrollable ways.

Both approaches react to current trends dominating the way infectious diseases are, or ought to be, perceived. Whittaker deals with the elements that make up the tropes and stories constantly renewing our fear and anxiety of infectious diseases, by engaging in a form of positive extrapolation: tropes and narratives about the significance of transmission are reframed into an intimate dimension that invite us to reflect on, question, and re-dress them, rather than just accepting them as universal. Although engaging in this game of repetition herself, by turning some of the objects displayed in her installations into modular items that recur across other exhibitions, Whittaker refuses to submit to the bleak, homogenizing single interpretation of near-apocalypse or the one-dimensional experience that news media or social media bubbles seem to offer. As the objects included in her installations are both iconic and very personal to the artist, even engaging with sensitive and very personal family histories, so they could be for the spectators. By creating objects derived from her personal recollections and anxiety about infectious diseases, Whittaker opens her installation to alternative interpretations. Viewers are encouraged to draw on their personal memories of outbreak or their personal stories on infectious disease, rather than solely on a series of default bytes or prefabricated notions.

Elle Mehrmand and Micha Cárdenas's *Virus.Circus* stage their science fictional vision in a future that looks safer but bleaker. In their performances, we are asked to reflect on our actions: whether we decide to play it safe or to take major risks, we are faced with making choices that will result in various sacrifices: safety for us and for others will trump enjoyment, but risk may endanger us and our neighbors. This dilemma is very much a great source of emotional burden and anxiety.

7

Breaking the Binaries, Embracing the Viral

The way different individuals define their relationships with viruses depends on their personal experience. For instance, immunosuppressed individuals may not buy the idea that the unknown, especially when it comes in the form of exposure to, or the effects of a pathogen, can be risked or even welcomed; the degree of anxiety that a person living in an outbreak area may experience is not comparable to that felt by an individual located in a safe area. Furthermore, the reaction to computer malware depends upon the type of activities and transactions affected by it: the fact that antivirus companies radically modified their visual and practical approach to viral threats reflects their increasing diversification and changing perception. So, personal—or professional—responses always take place within larger contexts: social, geographical, political, disciplinary, etc. For instance, the perception of Ebola shifted to become a real threat to countries outside of Africa only when it had acquired potential for extra-continental dissemination. The reaction was stark and immediate, prompting the closure of borders and the introduction of travel bans (Koch 2011). As noted, the perception of proximity and immediate threat has intensifying effects. This sort of reaction is also true when one considers natural disasters and other seemingly unpredictable phenomena (floods and eruptions occurring far away simply matter less than does a natural disaster that threatens the individual's immediate safety or livelihood).

This is also reflected in the way the artists and storytellers I described in the previous chapters have made decisions based on their personal histories and on their relationship with viruses. The previous chapter closed with questions about the risks and the consequences individuals are willing to accept when confronting viral phenomena. In this chapter, I want to push the notion of the viral further: to what degree, how, and in what circumstances is/can the viral be embraced, either as part of an ongoing artistic work or as part of the journey of a group or an individual? What if we decided to acknowledge the unpredictable outcome of viruses? What if we learnt how to cope with the capricious nature of these phenomena? This does not mean to accept one's fate or to declare defeat in front of a naturally occurring or partially controllable phenomenon. It is, instead, an invitation to search for a different *modus vivendi* able to coexist with those partial, complex, and multifaceted phenomena that cannot be captured or understood in their totality, nor perceived in universal ways.

My interest in finding ways to embrace the viral, or even to become viral, should not be interpreted as an invitation to passively accept it, or as a new form of fatalism. It is part of a search for ways to cope with the complexities of "incalculable" and apparently unpredictable events. Lacking strategies to flesh out these events in traditional ways, we must now turn to other methods, and what better method than to embody some of the qualities of the most resilient entities existing on earth? For some artists and practitioners, becoming viral may constitute a way to make a statement, to express concepts that cannot be expressed otherwise. For others, it is a necessity and a form of survival that later turns into a new way of existence and thriving. So, what does it mean to go viral?

The Provisional and Beyond

"Provisionality" is a common denominator in outbreaks and pandemics, computer network disruptions, and it can be seen, too, in their socio-cultural impacts. Manifesting in myriad ways, this quality is associated with the ever-changing knowledge about viruses: viruses are presented/seen as invisible (too small, too immaterial) and associated with unknown threats (the product of a lack of expertise or instruments). This quality endorses, simultaneously, differing positions, which present viruses as either threats or mere annoyances, as either entities to be feared, or as challenges to be conquered. Provisionality, not certainty, is the prevailing condition whenever there are attempts to describe, visualize, control, or warn about viruses: as accurate as these attempts appear to be, they are, in fact, mostly approximations, used to provide temporary solutions, patches to recurring complications, requiring constant adjustments as viruses morph, as they evolve, and as old versions recur or new ones emerge.

Fear may be triggered by several factors, but it can be shaped to benefit particular interests, for instance, to achieve a specific goal or to obtain some (political or financial) gains. The difficulty of predicting the spread of viruses leads to erratic responses when authorities make decisions to enhance security, surveillance, and monitoring systems to "manage" and "protect" the population against potential viral or security risks of various forms. However, it is the very lingering of a threat that has the potential to—yet it is not certain to—cause a great deal of damage, not the threat in itself, that produces fear and authorizes fearmongering and the deployment of all sorts of security measures (Massumi 2005; Ross 1991).

Provisionality is not (or not only) to be attributed to scientific or technological failure to delimit and contain viruses. If we were to call this a failure, we should blame the Cartesian system of thinking and its eternal search for closure and definite answers. In *The Hitchhikers' Guide to the Galaxy*, Douglas Adams humorously described science's quest for control and its constant search for exactitude. In the story, a supercomputer is built to calculate "the real answer to life, universe and everything" (Adams 1995). To an anxious crowd that had gathered to hear the answer, the computer responds: "42." The answer sounds disappointing. It provides a closure, but it does not explicate its rationale, nor does this ultimate number provide any real tangible certainty that people can understand. It is a number detached from its context. The scene humors the obsession of contemporary culture with finding the ultimate answer, and its feeling that things are even better if this answer is a number. However, it also resonates with contemporary culture: on the one hand, the practice of gathering concrete information that can be quantified produces the perception that more means better and more accurate results. On the other hand, it produces increasing dissatisfaction, as the search for precise data intensifies with further technological development and data increase; in the end, this endless revision of results produces more doubts about the validity of research. Data become unstable and unsatisfactory.

Having to deal with constantly changing and often contradictory data and provisional results can be paralyzing. Being affected by environmental changes, animal and human migrations, fast technological progress, the complexities of human/machine communication, viruses are deeply entangled with the context they inhabit and traverse, making it impossible to predict their status, their trajectories, and their transformations with certitude. This is the same sort of frustration that many complex phenomena evoke today. In his book *The Great Derangement*, Amitav Ghosh observes how freak events, flash storms, and other sudden shifts in the weather have recently become a more frequent occurrence in many parts of the world (Ghosh 2016). Climate change has made it increasingly difficult to predict atmospheric and seasonal changes. This has caused a growth in anxieties since the future can no longer be predicted using traditional tools. Our cultural and economic system is unable to adapt to this new normal, which is increasingly filled with what were once exceptions. The loss of perceived control resulting from this unpredictable new normal translates into an inability to cope and even to speak of it: our current literary, scientific, and storytelling traditions are not prepared to deal with such new paradigms (Ghosh 2016).

Rather than producing that sense of paralyzing fear so convenient for many parties involved in its management and modulation, provisionality can be interpreted as a challenge, and as a recurring condition that we should all be prepared to face; an event, or a series of events that we should learn how to handle; a sort of starting point for the formulation of a series of methodological moves and strategies for survival. So far, this book has illustrated how artists refuse to succumb to the paralyzing effects of provisionality by finding in it a strength or a source of energy. But can this proactive behavior be turned into a habitual approach to dealing with viral phenomena and newly emerging occurrences that escape any prediction?

Appropriating the Viral

The term viral is a powerful descriptor. It qualifies a few specific features that only apply to viruses. But it can also be used to label material qualities and behaviors beyond the territory of the biological and the informational. With the increase of Web usership, the use of the term viral to describe phenomena that only vaguely remind us of viruses has become common practice. Features that characterize viruses are applied to new phenomena (like viral marketing). Through a strangely uncontroversial process, these features are appropriated to describe phenomena whose dissemination is extraordinary and unexplained (like viral videos), expand quickly and through intricate networks. In this case, qualities that mark viruses' unique behavior are applied to other media phenomena. The term "going viral" is used when something (gossip, a message, a media campaign, an advertisement) is thought to be particularly effective in achieving goals such as increased dissemination and visibility, or improved awareness regarding a social or political issue.

Occurrences that happen to mimic one or more qualities of viruses are promptly associated with the attribute "viral." Among the millions of items being uploaded on a regular basis on social media platforms such as YouTube, Instagram, or TikTok, only a few reach exceptional, if unexpected, popularity. As Anna Munster argued in the previous chapter, there is no particular reason why certain videos would go viral and others would be completely ignored except for their communicability (Munster 2013). For Douglas Rushkoff, "the media virus is about us," not about the specific message it carries: titillating details draw us to certain scandalous and sensational content (Rushkoff 1996). Sound (a pleasant sound, a surprising voice) and colors (a familiar visual detail, a logo, etc.) are sufficient to produce "the viral." Outbreak narratives have gone viral because they contained clues, refrains, and symbols that sounded and resonated so well at the emotional and historical level.

By organizing, within the same expression, significant features common to viruses, the expanded use of the term viral produces divergent outcomes. Its use, or abuse, is symptomatic of an essentialist tendency that uses the "viral" as a sort of giant landfill-like space, in which one can throw anything pertaining to viruses. In fact, it appears to obliterate all possible differences that could help distinguish between the increasingly heterogeneous variety of multifunctional digital agents and "viral media."

This constitutes just one superficial facet of the viral—nonetheless an aspect that should not be ignored. As a catalyst of known qualities of viruses, the term viral is remarkably flexible. A viral infection is still very different from a viral network attack and is definitely not the same as media-based phenomena such as "viral marketing," "viral videos," and "viral tactics." Not only do these different phenomena engage different registers and operate via different communication codes (biology, computer language, media language, and/or cultural discourse), but they also affect distinct—yet somehow connected—environments (computer networks, human networks, media, and communication channels).

Media-based phenomena utilize the viral in quite different ways, as their level of engagement with, and mode of appropriation of various features and qualities borrowed from biological and computer viruses are substantially different. The emergence of phenomena that share the same suffix, and yet, interpret it in such different fashions, reveals that the viral should not be dismissed as "generalist" or "essentialist." In addition, it is true that viral media stem from popularly accepted characteristics from selected features of viruses, but these characteristics aggregate unevenly and crystallize to form different manifestations of the viral. Furthermore, the same characteristics can be applied to a diverse range of activities, thus leading to the formulation of a reservoir of tactics and actions.

The above double articulation of the "viral," as a term appropriated for specific applications (often leading to essentialist interpretations of viruses) and as an open-ended term, sheds a new light on expressions such as "viral marketing," "viral media," and "viral tactics." These expressions designate phenomena that originate from and owe their principal characteristics to viruses, and, thus, could not exist without them. In fact, although these viral phenomena are "other" than viruses, they cannot be separated (or not separated entirely) from them, as they emanate simultaneously as response to their current activity (viral media) and as contribution to their future—human-made—transformation (viral marketing). The aleatory and unpredictable behavior of viruses and their provisional nature in a sense allow for creative exploitation and appropriation of the features, name, and assumptions that define them.

Viruses of course are part of, and contributors to, a discourse that unifies computer viruses and biological viruses, their networks, their technological solutions and media channels, and their communities. Understanding the meaning of viruses through the frequent generalizations made about them, the creative interpretations made of their form and nature, and the appropriations of these help pinpoint and map how novel phenomena may emerge and manifest.

One may notice how many of these—brilliant and ingenious—new interpretations and uses that appropriate and exploit certain qualities of the viral to fit specific agendas are by nature opportunistic. These practices often appear to handpick those unique elements that distinguish viral entities and make them surprisingly effective; they are not necessarily motivated by a desire to explore different approaches to the viral, but to exploit viral features for their gain; they are not interested in uncovering different qualities of viruses through non-conventional interactions, but to achieve specific goals or sensationalistic effects by re-purposing their well-known, most peculiar or anxiety-inducing features; they are not committed to acknowledging and reflecting on the multiple connections, the intersections, the cross-disciplinary engagements that viruses engage in, through the viral. The viral is, under these circumstances, turned into a tool, a device that can be manipulated to achieve a specific goal, not a concept, a set of behaviors to think or interact with.

Using terminology that directly references viruses has become a strategy to draw more attention from the media. This is certainly the case of viral marketing. Commercial enterprises and marketing companies quickly noticed the effectiveness of viral media and proceeded to re-purpose the qualities enabling items to circulate and go viral to produce specific results. Their purpose was to strip viruses of their negative connotations and transform their impressive productivity to benefit themselves or those who employ them.

Viral marketing is often described as "the tactic of 'creating a process where interested people can market to each other'" (Subramani and Rajagopalan 2003). Drawing on the insights of information process theory, Subramani and Rajagopalan classify this tactic as a specific manifestation of the "more general phenomenon of knowledge-sharing and influence among individuals in social networks" (301). The first commercial "viral marketing" campaigns were introduced in the 1940s (Rosen 2000). However, the label viral has only recently been applied to the specific marketing tactics introduced on the internet. The new denomination would not have been adopted had there not been an acknowledgment of the benefits that this new formula would generate. Clearly, "viral marketers" know that using the term viral draws a great deal of publicity. In addition to reminding one of the resemblances between this marketing tactic and the spread of computer and biological viruses, the term appears to have been adopted to achieve an augmented ability for the dissemination and penetration of new markets and the pockets of interested parties.

A case in point is the use of the viral to launch daring marketing campaigns for the entertainment industry: the 1999 campaign for the movie *The Blair Witch Project* is a case in point. The promotion of this film constituted one of the first attempts at viral marketing spread by "word-of-mouse" (Boase and Wellman 2001; Subramani and Rajagopalan 2003). A low-budget, supernatural horror, *The Blair Witch Project* is thought to be the first widely released film marketed primarily by the internet (Weinraub 1999). While the movie did not achieve a great success at the box office, its marketing campaign exceeded all expectations; it successfully used the potential of the then pre-web 2.0 medium of the worldwide web to build excitement about the movie among young internet explorers and effectively became the first campaign to go viral (Bowls 2014).

The movie, produced, directed, and edited on a minimal budget by Daniel Myrick and Eduardo Sanchez, plays with the concepts of fiction and reality by pretending to be a documentary created from "found footage" left by three young filmmakers who had disappeared in the woods of Maryland. The story is obviously fictional, but by tapping into very real fears and using real locations as evidence, the film managed to make the story seem real for many people, including the police.

The movie opened the door to a new marketing practice. Following the success of the film's promotional campaign, many other viral campaigns have been created. This time, feasibility studies and statistical data preceded the campaigns, to determine strategies to maximize dissemination, thus making virality predictable. Digital-native millennials, who lead social media-rich lives, seek principles that make media go viral in order to build their online personas and social status (*Generation Like* [2014]).

The term viral has also been associated with specific forms of media activism. Viral tactics, an expression coined by Nathan Martin during a speech delivered at the festival of tactical media Next Five Minutes in 2003, has since become a common term used to label a certain mode of activism used by tactical media practitioners that spreads quickly across many networks and produces some action (Martin 2003). Unfortunately, viral tactics, originally meant to create media noise, or to shake mainstream news, has recently gone hand in hand with the spread of fake news too, and such tactics have been appropriated by those who spread misinformation and disinformation.

Shao et al. note how viral content (i.e., content meant to go viral), especially in the form of "misleading news reports, hoaxes, conspiracy theories, click-bait headlines, junk science, and even satire" can successfully exploit cognitive, social, and cultural "vulnerabilities," and influence public opinion. This ability is intensified "thanks to the low cost of producing fraudulent websites and high volumes of software-controlled profiles, known as social bots misinformation" (Shao et al. 2018). The motives for and the benefits of this type of game are not only financial, but also political: Shao et al. observed that since around 2010, "influential bots have affected online debates about vaccination policies, and participated actively in political campaigns, both in the United States and other countries" (Shao et al. 2018). Interestingly, the spread of infectious diseases, such as Ebola, and the recent COVID-19 pandemic have become very fertile grounds for viral media and viral tactics in the forms of outbreak narratives, calls for action, and, sadly, fake news and conspiracy theories. In other words, the virus turned on itself and went viral. Viruses turned out to be not only structurally and behaviorally provisional, but also susceptible to network and media volatility.

Taming the Viral

Considering the success of "everything going viral," one might think that viruses, whether they are the causes of infectious diseases, whether they exist as malware that bring down distributed networks, or constitute particular types of communication, work well, as their somehow controlled imitation demonstrates. If controlling the viral is so successful, then, why are viral events mostly described as unprecedented or exceptional, as accidents, as atypical/unexplained moments, or as networks considered out of control?

Galloway and Thacker, in their analysis of network culture, mentioned that one of the common assumptions regarding viruses is that they appear to "spiral out of control" (Galloway and Thacker 2007, 5). This is not the case, however. "[C]alling such instances 'accidents' or networks 'out of control' is a misnomer. They are not networks that are somehow broken, but *networks that work too well*. They are networks beyond one's capacity to control them, or even comprehend them" (6). The contraposition between distributed networks and the need to control them is an expression of the "clash" between materiality and design, sovereignty and structure (Galloway and Thacker 2007). In other words, the way viruses behave or spread, the way they exist in nature, because of their inherent material features, conflicts with the attempt to control and dominate them. As Esposito argued in Chapter 3, either politics attempt to domesticate life (*biós*) to fit rules and categories, or life and its irreducible complexity eternally escape these rules (Esposito 2008). The distributed and unpredictable spread that characterizes not only biological viruses, but also their computer kin makes it hard to control them. Clearly, issues of control, binary thinking, and anthropocentric opportunism are at stake here.

Acknowledgment of the advantages that taming this "out-of-controlness" can bring is at the core of many attempts to appropriate the viral. However, once launched, a virus can only be partially controlled. We know now from past and present epidemics and outbreaks that there does not exist a fit-all solution or a certain infallible behavior to stopping a virus, and that each geographical area, population conglomerate, online network, and cultural enclosure will have the power to change, often inexplicably, their course. Likewise, although viral marketing and viral tactics can be launched to obtain a particular goal, the outcomes of these schemes are difficult to predict, as they can produce unexpected results. For viral marketing, a certain margin of unpredictability can constitute a risk, as not reaching the projected goals may negatively affect sales or hinder the penetration of a certain demographic.

This situation poses a major dilemma for those media practitioners involved in activism that tries to oppose hegemonic socioeconomic structures. In order to improve their visibility and have their voice heard, these individuals and groups often have no other option but to operate outside of predictable behavioral patterns and conventions. What if, for instance, a particular action does not result in a desired outcome? What if instead of helping a cause, it backfired horribly, jeopardizing the safety of vulnerable groups? This is a dilemma that was often discussed in early tactical media and current activist circles. In fact, one criticism that has often been directed at the almost spontaneous guerrilla interventions characterizing Tactical Media is the fact that they are often temporary and lack a well-defined and comprehensive strategy of action. In other words, like a virus, practitioners can cause—sometimes very effective—small outbreaks that might temporarily stop harmful corporate activities, or exploitative labor conditions or other urgent injustices (Critical Art Ensemble 2008; Martin 2008).

This practice was particularly popular at the end of the 1990s, but it became less widespread in the following decade. However, tactical media practitioners are still very active, acting quickly and autonomously, planting seeds of dissent that can either flourish beautifully or be killed horribly, using media jamming and disruption, revealing the inner functioning of media and algorithmic machineries, or the endless wave of "artificial stupidity" perpetuated by mainstream media and the users' blind acceptance of it (Yetiskin 2014). Because of their provisional and uncertain nature, tactical media have often been deemed ineffective, short-lived or humorous, or a wasteful activity.

When they work, however, viral tactics have gifted us some of the best and most effective pranks in the past decades: the humorous and disruptive actions of the Yes Men are well-known examples of what can be achieved at the expense of multinational corporate power, such as Dow Chemicals, ExxonMobil, and the WTO (Reilly 2013)[1]. These actions contribute to a constant revision and reconfiguration of the way media and capital conglomerates are conceived, understood, and used. These revisions bring molecular, often imperceptible changes, but changes, nonetheless. Generally, the success of activism and antagonist media is assessed in terms of the outcomes and the changes they can achieve. The very process of going viral (the process leading to mobilization, the formulation of tactics to use, the

[1]The Yes Men have been known for impersonating corporate representatives and hijacking panels and conferences, calling fake press releases and giving fake interviews. The Yes Men targeted the WTO in various occasions by creating a fake website and accepting engagements and interviews from misled officials on behalf of the WTO. Their speeches ranged from admitting to unethical and careless practices to absurd proposals. The Dow Chemical prank was perpetrated at the expenses of Dow Chemicals/Union Carbide on the twentieth anniversary of the Bhopal disaster. Andy Bichlbaum delivered an interview with BBC impersonating a Dow Chemical announcing their responsibility in the disaster and their desire to compensate the victims. At Canada's largest oil conference, they posed as Exxonmobil representatives, admitting that the current oil operations ".. are increasing the chances of huge global calamities. But … in the worst-case scenario, the oil industry could 'keep fuel flowing' by transforming the billions of people who would die into oil."

organizing needed to make something go viral), the relational aspects of it (the way communities come together, the analysis of what "sticky" elements have enabled the viral process), the speed, and the extent of dissemination are usually dismissed. This tendency is telling; it speaks of a general inability to think beyond linear narratives, narratives linked to precise goals and expected outcomes, assessed against a set of anticipations and measurable projections.

Linear ways of thinking (i.e., I do this to achieve that) are inadequate when trying to understand and establish a dialogue with the viral. Yet, as the prevailing narratives confirm, they still constitute the preferred way of assessing its effects and successes. Of course, these ways of thinking fail to render the truth of viruses' (and viral media) entanglement with the surrounding environment, their extraordinary propagation across disciplines, their liminal nature and provisional behavior. In the medical sciences, and to a certain extent in computer science, studies have demonstrated the complex ways in which viruses interact with and intersect with diverse environments. Viruses reside pretty much everywhere, even in places, like Antarctica, that were deemed free of them since relatively recently. In the ocean, they outnumber all other residents by fifteen to one. Viruses can be found in the human genome, which contains genes from 30 million years ago. Their ubiquitous existence and their utility merits are quite obvious (Cobián Güemes et al. 2016; Zimmer 2015; 2021). However, in the presence of medical emergencies such as an infectious disease outbreaks, or in cases of major network disruptions, the idea of viruses as disruptors and evil attackers seems to resurface and prevail once again.

The (mis)understanding of the viral and the resulting use of viral metaphors perpetuate a tradition (saturated, as it has been noticed elsewhere, with centuries of scientific and popular rhetoric) that directly connects viruses to disruption and malfunctioning. The same rhetoric extends across all instances of the viral and affects current research involving the material being and manipulation of viruses. The bad rep of viruses combined with the outcome-driven nature of research encouraged by institutions and funding schemes makes it unlikely to call a virus "useful," "good," or "benevolent."

This difficulty was discussed at great length in the computer science and computer security community in the 1980s, against voices that defended computer viruses and worms' identity as forms of artificial life or as forms with the ability to improve the state and the quality of networks (John Aycock and Maurushat 2008; Bontchev 1994; F. B. Cohen 1991; Ludwig 1995; Sampson 2005). In the medical and immunological field, new practices such as the experimental immune therapy involving the use of oncolytic viruses—viruses found in nature as well as viruses modified in the laboratory—to target tumors or other diseases have caused some to see the utility, the "good" of viruses. However, while acknowledging the pervading ability of viruses as crucial in the successful delivery of the therapy, researchers are very cautious to explain the process of manipulating and engineering them, and to confirm their official approval by the food and drug administration or other institutions before they can be inserted successfully in the body of the patient (Bell et al. 2002; Kelly and Russell 2007). Phage therapy, an early version of immune therapy, employs viruses that eat bacteria (literally bacterio-phage) to defeat bacterial infections. Practiced in the early twentieth century, its use was later supplanted when the use of antibiotics became more widespread. This "forgotten cure" was the victim of medical politics and Cold War power dynamics, two aspects that did not help its wide dissemination (Kuchment 2011).

In all cases, the acknowledgment that viruses may be accomplishing very useful tasks always implies that in order to be useful viruses must directly benefit humans or must have positively contributed to their development as a species. In order to do that, the intervention of human agency as catalyst for the transformation of a virus into a good virus or the discovery of a good virus is needed.

In Search of the Good Virus

Computer virus researcher Fred Cohen famously argued that "good computer viruses" could be a possibility (Cohen 1991). Computer viruses, he maintained, could technically perform a series of useful operations. Cohen offered a reward of $1,000 to anyone able to present him with a useful virus. Unfortunately, his call has not been fulfilled yet. The problem here, as a popular (and maybe unique) paper by Bulgarian computer analyst Vasselin Bontchev stated, has technical, ethical, and psychological ramifications (Bontchev 1994). In fact, as Aykock and Maurushat confirm, one could technically create a useful *human right worm* aimed at automatically testing the state of a censorship system (the two authors mention China). However, this activity is not only dangerous, but also illegal (John Aycock and Maurushat 2008).

One of the main reasons that prevent computer scientists from creating a "good virus" is the stigma and the assumptions that accompany it. For Cohen, a benevolent virus can be placed alongside malware, or, as John Aycock calls it, using the oxymoron "benevolent malware," "software which would otherwise be classified as malware, yet is intended to have good effects" (Critical Art Ensemble 2008, 177; Martin 2008).

Bontchev agrees that it is possible to target and neutralize malware by launching ad hoc counterviruses (Aycock 2006; Bontchev 1994; Sampson 2005). In other words,

> Declaring some viruses as 'good' and 'beneficial' would just provide an excuse to the crowd of irresponsible virus writers to condone their activities and to claim that they are actually doing some kind of 'research.' In fact, this is already happening—the people mentioned above are often

> quoting Dr. Fred Cohen's ideas for beneficial viruses as an excuse of what they are doing—often without even bothering to understand what Dr. Cohen is talking about.
>
> (Bontchev 1994)

For many, invoking the "goodness" of a particular virus or worm is just an unconvincing excuse to legitimize the spread of more malware. This excuse did not help early virus writers such as Sven Jaschan, the German teenager behind the creation of the "*Sasser worm*," for instance, who claimed his innocence by confessing that he had fabricated different variants to neutralize the original worm (TrendlabsResearch 2004). He admitted to having also been the author of a few variants of Netsky, a worm that attempted to neutralize other families of worms: respectively, "Mydoom" and "Bagle" (known also as "Bagel"). Nor was Robert Morris Jr. excused for freeing his infamous computer worm across the internet on November 2, 1988, causing a series of denial-of-service attacks, but later claiming that his goal was not to create damage. While the worm served some good in that it helped to reveal several network vulnerabilities, the news media and authorities decided to focus on the illegal nature of the security breaches caused by the worm and on the potential for future attacks that the work could enable, as well as on the damage (mostly measured in slowdowns and inconveniences) it caused. The incident confirmed the obsessive attention of government and industry for network threats in a society increasingly dependent on computer networks to function and to make transactions. The fact that it was a student, not a professional, who had been able to temporarily jam the network made it even more urgent to make an example out of the accident (Parikka 2007). This situation called for a confirmation of the dangerous qualities of viruses, certainly not the opposite.

Following these incidents, there have been numerous discussions about the malevolent nature of computer viruses and worms. Bontchev (1994) casts his doubts on the possibility that a truly benevolent malware could be created. Serious experiments to launch "predator worms" that target specific malware have not been successful. There are problems of control (once a worm is released, the person who released it has no control on how it will spread), compatibility (there is a question of how many worms should be launched and how effective would they be against different strains), and the "thorny issue of verification" (how can users know that they are not dealing with a false benevolent malware? And how can they know how this type of virus will behave once in their computers? How can the antivirus company have the user's trust?). Finally, he admits that the antivirus industry is not in the position to call any service a "beneficial virus" or benevolent malware, as users would not give them permission to install it on their system. Due to the bad reputation of viruses, users just would not believe that they could be turned into a beneficial service (Bontchev 1994).

The early debate about the existence and the use of "benevolent malware" not only illustrates the challenges of employing a virus for useful reasons and still call it a virus. It also demonstrates the assumption that virus writers cannot produce any virus with positive/helpful qualities. Defining malware as "benevolent" is made impossible both by historical conventions and by the very role it plays in popular imagination. The latest generation of malware has confirmed and solidified these assumptions: the emergence of spyware and the most recent ransomware, which penetrates computer systems to gather personal/sensitive information or to blackmail the user for personal gain, has certainly not helped dissipate them.

The Good Virus: With a Little Help from Human Friends

There seems to be a general agreement that benevolent pathogens and good computer viruses are hard to find or to fabricate. Biological viruses are usually classified according to the kind of immune response they receive from a host. This approach ends up prioritizing the impact on humans and on other animals in contact with or participating in the sustenance of human beings. As a result, disproportionate attention is given to viruses that make us sick. The attention shifts to other viruses when human agency intervenes to exploit or turn a virus into a benevolent one. Although it was not until the 1940s that Barbara McClintock discovered transposition, demonstrating how genes could turn physical characteristics on and off in plants, earlier attempts to obtain such results can be found as early as the seventeenth century. "Tulipmania" was a fascinating case of intense speculation on the sale of tulips, involving a virus (a "tulip breaking virus"), able to introduce a mutation resulting in desirable appearance. Botanist Dag-Ragnar-Blystad observes that viruses such as *tulip breaking virus* and *abutilon mosaic virus* are often responsible for giving plants a particularly interesting and pleasant appearance without necessarily reducing their longevity and productivity. These plants are often coveted and purposely infected in order to increase sales (Blystad 2020). The industry producing Genetically Modified plants is not unfamiliar with the use of viruses; many GM plants are engineered to contain a promoter from the Cauliflower Mosaic Virus (CaMV) in order to facilitate expression of an engineered target gene (Bak and Emerson 2020).

The above examples show how naturally occurring viruses have contributed to benefit people's businesses, enhance the enjoyment of plants, and label products. These approaches are all the result of anthropocentric views that elevate the role of the human as virus handler. Human intervention here is seen as instrumental in directing a virus toward accomplishing specific tasks that will benefit human activities and well-being. No self-replicating program (whether aspiring to be benevolent or not) can be left to roam freely across networks to create potential unexpected situations; however, human interference will help it to fulfill tasks that will improve a system's performance and productivity, be it in the biological or informational realm. Such view of human agency can be found in the development of two emerging (or rediscovered) therapies in the realm of immunology: the re-habilitation and further development of phage therapy and the use of oncolytic viruses in drug delivery. In both cases, agency and control, as well as their relations with global politics and economic imperatives, have played crucial roles in shaping their spread and in paving their successes.

In her history on phage therapy, Anna Kuchment narrates the trajectory of phage therapy from—literally—riches to rags, and possibly back to riches again (Bak and Emerson 2020; Kuchment 2011). From being considered a revolutionary and even miraculous cure against mortal bacterial infections such as peritonitis or dysentery, phage therapy was demoted to become an obscure and supposedly unreliable remedy. The popularity of phage research and phage therapy, according to Kuchment's account, spans just over thirty years, between 1917 and the mid-1940s with the beginning of the Cold War.

A bacteriophage is a small bacteria-eating virus, a microorganism "developing at the expense of" (3) bacteria, as Felix d'Herelle described them in 1917. Under an electron microscope "bacteriophages look like insects from outer space. They have a round, polyhedral head, elongated bodies, a tail, and spindly, spiderlike legs" (xi). Carl Zimmer describes them as "some lunar space landing modules" (*Viruses are Everywhere!* (2011)). Often confused, especially because of their alien visual form, with the viruses affecting mammals, these pathogens target bacteria instead: they inject their DNA into the cell of bacteria, "shutting down the cell's reproductive machinery and reprogramming it to make phages instead of bacteria" (Kuchment 2011, xii). Once they have filled the bacteria, phages exit it by bursting its walls, hence destroying it.

Although very promising, and for a certain period flourishing as a medical practice, Kuchment argues that phage therapy was supplanted in the 1940s by the discovery of penicillin and by the rise of the antibiotic industry. The later neglect and abandonment of phage therapy had both economic and political motivations. Because each phage is unique to the bacteria affecting an individual patient, microbiologists must spend time in the lab identifying and matching the bacteria in their tissue sample with the right phage. Thus, phages are at the most effective when used to treat chronic ailments, rather than acute conditions. Economically speaking, this process was considered wasteful, especially when it became evident that antibiotics offered relatively quick resolutions in a much higher number of patients. Phage therapy was not efficient enough in curing infections. Politically speaking, internal conflicts within the scientific community, d'Herelle's alleged difficult personality, his early involvement with the Russian Communist party, and the succeeding Cold War sanctioned the abandonment of phage therapy in the West, where antibiotics became the preferred method of treatment, and the continued extensive use of the therapy in the Eastern bloc. It is not surprising that Tbilisi, in former Soviet republic of Georgia, hosts a major center for the study of phage therapy.

Literally forgotten for decades, phage therapy was rediscovered in the West in the mid-1990s, when it not only became evident that antibiotics were losing their effectiveness against bacterial infections, but that they have become increasingly scarce, as pharmaceutical companies had unwisely made the decision to focus their efforts on producing more lucrative drugs for chronic diseases such as diabetes and high blood pressure rather than continuing their research on antibiotics (*Viruses are Everywhere!* (2011)). Phage treatment, which had been deemed unviable and financially unsustainable, was becoming sexy again.

The renewed attention was only in part caused by an interest in the potentials of phages. Recent genetic engineering development has been responsible for bringing "a steady stream of venture capitalists, entrepreneurs and physicians through the Eliava Institute's halls" (Kuchment 2011, xiii). Whether led by the scientific and medical urge to find an alternative to a remedy that had an expiry date on it, by a surge of interest in the importance of the human microbiota (Malik et al. 2017), or by the financially lucrative opportunities that exploiting this emergency would bring (a particular type of disaster capitalism), these individuals saw in phages many opportunities indeed.

But there is another reason why phage therapy was largely abandoned in the West. Perceived problems of control resulted in phage therapy being seen as an unreliable cure that could not be completely trusted. During a podcast interview, Carl Zimmer wonders why the FDA has been reluctant to approve the use of phages for therapeutic purposes. In part, he says, this is because phages are viruses. Besides their controversial reputation, it is believed that viruses' ability to mutate easily makes them unreliable: "Much of the difficulty in obtaining regulatory approval [to pursue phage therapy] is proving to be the risks of using a self-replicating entity which has the capability to evolve." In fact, as antibiotics' action is relatively stable (when it works), since they destroy the bacteria that cause diseases, and fast, this is not the case with phages. Phage therapy doesn't always work as expected and sometimes requires more trials before it succeeds. In addition, there is always a risk that certain groups of phages may promote, rather than halt, the exchange of DNA among bacteria, as in the case of cholera, making them stronger and causing an exacerbation of the outbreak.

According to Charlotte Brives (2021), who has studied bacteriophage and phage therapy extensively, the issues at stake pertain both to the understanding of "therapy," and to the interpretation of what phages are and do. In fact, the assumption that we can apply the same technique to entire sections of the population affected by similar ailments, that is, that there exists a medicine that fits all, is still widely accepted. This very assumption is well demonstrated by the popularity of antibiotics, considered powerful and almost universal remedies for infections that don't need to be exactly and individually diagnosed. However, Brives observes, our relation with microorganisms is complex and situated. She defines this relationship as Pluribiosis, or the "recognition of the existence of multiple relational spectra between entities forever in the process of becoming, constantly shaped and transformed by their interactions with other living things, and by the context in which they occur" (2). Because of this complex relationality involving humans, microorganisms, and different situated environments, phage therapy cannot be considered a universal solution, but "offers us narratives that refuse fixity" and forces us to "recognise the situated knowledge and situated biologies, and therefore the necessarily situated character, of their applications in biomedicine" (3).

In a way, a push in this direction can be observed in the interest of biotech companies to study ways of using phages that are genetically engineered to "use a DNA editing system called CRISPR to kill only antibiotic resistant bacteria" (Reardon 2014). Their motivation seems to match, in reverse, the reason why phage therapy was rejected in the first place in favor of antibiotics. If antibiotics seemed to be initially the best choice, because of their immediate effectiveness, now the ability of new genetic engineering techniques to manipulate and precisely direct phages to target bad bacteria promises even more control over the process and the results of a therapy. Microbiologist Michael Schmidt describes the growing appreciation that "wiping out the human body's beneficial microbes along with disease-causing ones can create a niche in which antibiotic-resistant bacteria can thrive." "Antibiotics are a big hammer," Schmidt says. "You want a guided missile" (Reardon 2014), which is exactly what a microorganism modified and improved to contain targeted weapons is.

As the fight against diseases becomes more sophisticated, the medical field is called upon to develop increasingly precise, controllable, and reliable therapeutic strategies. Emerging oncoimmunotherapy, for instance, has been showing such great promise and has been hailed by some as a solution that might supplant much hated and generally aggressive chemotherapy. Although such therapies are new, the medical and immunology fields have been attracted to the potentials of viruses as possible agents of tumor destruction for a long time. At the end of the nineteenth century, medical professionals observed that, occasionally, cancer patients who had contracted an infectious disease such as influenza were experiencing a brief period of clinical remission. In a 1896 well-documented case, a doctor observed a dramatic improvement in a woman affected by leukemia who had contracted influenza (Kelly and Russell 2007). The observation is even more remarkable when one considers that the existence and nature of viruses were formalized over thirty years later. This case made researchers wonder whether it could be possible to offer cancer patients a virus with attenuated pathogenic effects and enhanced cancer-killing potency. In fact, experiments on rodents showed promises, but the short-lived improvements produced by the administered viruses were often accompanied by high morbidity rates. In sum, while the virus cancer-killing qualities of the virus would improve the patients' conditions, its pathogenic qualities could likely kill them.

Numerous attempts through the 1950s and 1960s followed to force the evolution of viruses with greater tumor specificity, with famous and infamous attempts: for instance, in Japan, the paramyxovirus mumps—a pathogen used initially to stimulate the immune system of patients not responding to traditional cancer treatments—was used to perform virotherapy. In the United States, Dr. Chester Southam used the West Nile virus as a pathogen with milder potency. His experiments went out of hand when he enlisted jail prisoners and the elderly as his guinea pigs, injecting them with cancer cells purposely to study the immune response to cancer (Sepkowitz 2009).

Virotherapy briefly employed animal viruses as attenuated versions of human pathogens in an attempt to reduce the morbidity triggered by the cure, but it was only when bioengineering made the modification, adaptation, and attenuation of viruses possible that oncolytic viruses became really popular in the biomedical community. Thanks to developments in bioengineering, bioinformatics, and synthetic biology, today's oncoimmunotherapy uses human viruses that are deactivated and made innocuous. For instance, bioengineering has allowed the use of HIV viruses with "attenuate[d] pathogenicity, increase[d] oncolytic potency, or enhance[d] specificity for cancer tissue" (Kelly and Russell 2007). The first marketing approval of an oncolytic virus is relatively recent and was granted by Chinese regulators for the genetically modified oncolytic adenovirus H101 in November 2005 (Bell et al. 2002). Shortly after, a fast proliferating industry of biotech start-ups with more or less commercial intents has flourished. Specializing in immunotherapy and oncoimmunotherapy research and collaborating with major pharmaceutical companies, companies such as Oncorus ("Oncorus" n.d.), and PsiOxus ("PsiOxus Therapeutics Home—PsiOxus Therapeutics" n.d.) have been busy experimenting oncolytic viruses therapies to treat cancer currently in clinical testing.

The story of oncolytic viruses should give pause for reflection. On the one hand, the interest in more personalized forms of therapies acknowledges the complex relationships between humans, microorganisms, and the environment described by Brives, and reflects a need to move away from standardized medicine to focus on more personalized, situated solutions. On the other hand, the drive to modify, adapt, and ultimately fabricate a virus that fits human needs is the product of a typical anthropocentric narrative. Viruses, in this narrative, appear useful when and if they can be used for human's benefits. While viruses may be seen as able to deliver some surprising benefits, this potential, it's usually believed, can only be exploited through human intervention and domestication. The molecular engineering of specific functions of viruses is constellated with extreme daring and a good dose of human hubris: here one can see scenes of tentative experimentation with an entity still unknown but manifesting strange pharmakon-like qualities that can cure a lethal disease if it could only be properly directed.

The desire to explore all routes in an effort to "bend" viruses to humans' will has been driven by a trust in the eventual success of human intervention. For instance, today's fascination for hacking and bio-hacking has brought an overconfidence in the ability to re-program viruses just like a computer hacker would re-program a software to perform according to their needs. This has brought bio-hacker/entrepreneur like Andrew Hassel to downplay the difficulties in fabricating oncolytic viruses with the following statement: "You can do the design on computers—something I was very familiar with in bioinformatics—and then print the DNA" (de Lange 2014). In addition, the early discoveries of the potentially healing values of certain viruses led to taking substantial risks and to making inconsiderate and often-cruel decisions that often sacrificed other people's lives, all lives deemed unworthy of saving because they were seen as already desperately compromised or corrupted to start with. Even today, the race to develop oncolytic viruses is driven by the partial success of traditional pharmaceutical remedies and by the fact that many patients being recommended oncolytic virotherapy are at the proverbial "end of the rope."

Viruses and Co-Dependency

The experimentation and use of oncolytic viruses also tell a different story. Research on virotherapy could suggest, as Brives explains, new ways "to think beyond the old dichotomy of the living and non-living and instead to embrace a broader understanding of the fundamentally relational nature of biological entities" (Brives 2021). In fact, this research has led to a further acknowledgment of the similarities between human and animal pathogens and to a better understanding of kinship and mutual interdependence, a confirmation that viruses (or infectious diseases) are in a position of non-competing mutuality, co-construction, and co-existence, where "the natural world only acquires definite boundaries, and concepts only acquire definite content, together" (Rouse 2004, 149).

The now confirmed endosymbiotic theory formulated by Lynn Margulis is a radical departure from historical understanding of living systems: multicellular fungi and plants are supracellular assemblies as their cells are not physically separated from each other. There are also examples of alliances and merging between multicellular organisms. In this process, viral infections are considered major forces driving the biological evolution toward higher complexity (Baluska 2009). Margaret McFall Ngai observed how what we assumed to be a self-contained entity is actually a plurality of indivisible organisms in symbiosis with each other. Inspired by Lynn Margulis, she argues that organisms only survive and evolve thanks to other organisms living inside them or in close proximity to them: "every I is also a We" (McFall Ngai 2017). We can no longer think of living systems as self-contained and simplify them through one-fit-all models and formulas. "Tree of Life, Forest of Life, Web of Life, Mess of Life—What is it after all?" asks Eugene Koonin: traditional methods and taxonomic boxes that science used to rely on are increasingly difficult to fill (Puigbò, Wolf, Koonin 2013). This way of thinking re-inscribes humans and viruses in a co-dependent and even symbiotic relation where humans are interested in the complexity of these entities because of the benefits that each could bring to the other, and not solely for the anthropocentric benefits that can be gained from the exploitation of viruses in the name of human progress.

Since 2015, interdisciplinary artist and designer Pei-Ying Lin has been researching the relationship between human beings and viruses. During this long-term project, she engaged with virologists, humanists, and performers, building installations, assembling board games, staging video performances and group socials, as well as writing a cookbook where she asked recurring questions: How do humans coexist with their viruses? Is it possible to tame and domesticate a virus? Her speculative design narratives imagine futures where viruses are incorporated into everyday activities.

In *Smallpox Syndrome* (Figure 29), she imagines a future where biotechnology merges with the eastern philosophy around medicine: "Instead of combating the pathogens, the focus shift towards how to enhance human immune system for unpredicted infectious diseases" (Lin n.d.). Can we eat a virus, engage with it, and simulate its properties in order to become more resilient or more resistant to it, thus turning it into a non-threatening entity? Combining vaccine research and makeup, a vaccine is custom-programmed to be worn and displayed as a skin mark and as a fashion statement. In addition, different marks on the skin become an open declaration of the level of immunity of an individual as well as the degree to which the individual has engaged and co-evolved with the virus. A more recent performance, part of the a series of installations titled *Tame Is to Tame*, dancer and choreographer Hsin Yu Chang demonstrates special exercises to avoid contact with surfaces infected with a virus.

However, the sinuous and elegant moves of the dancer are neither aggressive nor fearful, as she appears to be dancing with the virus, gently avoiding the surfaces where it potentially hides, and using caution to be able to coexist side by side the virus, without trying to kill it, hide from it, or reject its existence.

For Pei-Ying Lin, "taming" is to acknowledge that viruses cannot be deleted. Since they are part of our daily life, they can be at least made familiar. This means to engage in a dance with an invisible entity that can be perceived but not seen (literally expressed through the performance *Tame Is to Tame*). The relationship with the viral expressed by Lin is not of domination, but coexistence. Viruses after all do not act alone in their interactions with other organisms but are always "produced by a multiplicity of relations" (Stengers 2011, 33). They are a part of the collectivity of other phenomena,

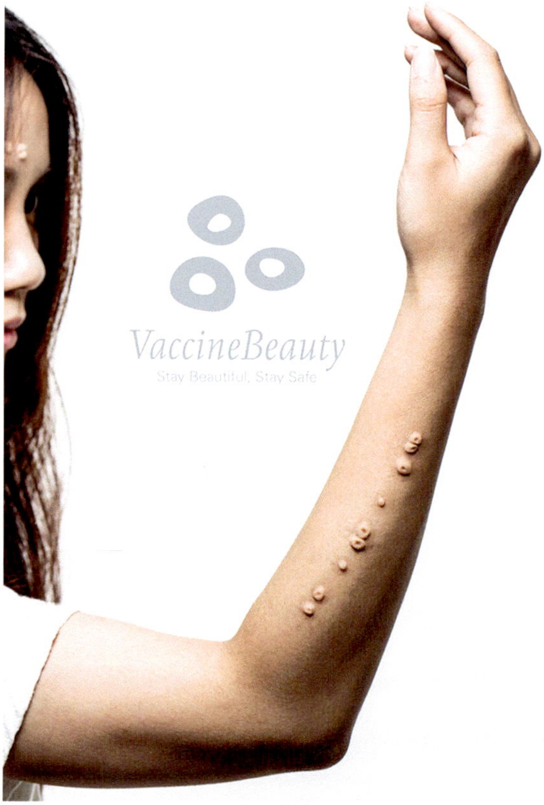

FIGURE 29 *Pei-Ying Lin,* Vaccine Beauty, *2016. © Pei-Ying Lin.*

individuals, and the environment that surround them and that, together, they create a condition of unavoidable reciprocity and coexistence.

This relationship can be applied to all forms of viral phenomena. The artists and collectives I will examine in the next pages show an open-minded approach to the potentials of the viral, to the multiplicity of relations contributing to its formation and circulation, and to the aleatory features of biological viruses and their computer counterparts. One important aspect emerges from these interventions: in all cases, openness toward viruses, whether informational or biological, was dictated by the curiosity to find out how far the viral would go, what opportunities it would bring about, and what new aesthetics it would generate. The alleged dangerous or vicious aspects of viruses were not just used to cause clamor, but also to draw attention to specific and important issues that would otherwise lie hidden. This is not to downplay the disruptive power of viruses or the suffering of those in the most vulnerable positions. However, in acknowledging such sufferings, I also want to give voice to alternative strategies to fight, exercise, embrace, or comprehend viruses. While some of these strategies may come from a position of privilege, others stem from a genuine necessity to apply a different lens and perspective to a series of phenomena that our current epistemologies have made only partially comprehensible.

Constructive Noise and *Viractual* Insights

Some artistic and media practices have acknowledged the viral as a force that needn't be tamed at any cost; instead, they have embraced it as a crucial part of the multiplicity of phenomena that can live and cross the boundaries of information and biology, medical sciences, popular science, and the arts. These practices, which go back respectively to the mid-1980s—at the height of the AIDS pandemic—and the beginning of the Millenium—just when computer viruses had become an important presence in the context of network culture—reflect different states and interpretations of what viruses represent for the human. To various degrees, and driven by radically different goals, Joseph Nechvatal and the duo 0100101110101101.org, known today as Eva and Franco Mattes, explored the ability of the viral to cross domains and media and to embrace its open-ended outcomes and its resistance to human control. They also explored viruses' entanglement with surrounding environments and nearby cultures, and their ability to transform these environments and cultures.

While reflecting on his long-term artistic practice working with digital items and real-world material objects, Joseph Nechvatal defined the term *viractual* as "a new topological cognitive vision of connection between the computed virtual and the un-computed corporeal world" (Nechvatal 2011). For Nechvatal, the *viractual* is the conscious convergence, the interface between the biological and the virtual. This definition very much aligns with the idea that information and biology, virtual and actual, biology and information do not lie in well-separated or unbridgeable containers, but are situated in a condition of mutual becoming, a "co-production or co-evolution of people and things" (Fishel 2017, 7).

Nechvatal's use of the *viractual* in his artistic practice is meant to reveal "the power of digitization while being culturally aware of the values of monumentality and permanency" (Nechvatal 2002). The emergence of the viral in the artist's work developed out of his search for a way to demonstrate how virtual and real may intersect and merge into each other: "When I began exploring the viractual image in 1986, I created ridiculously complex numeric images which consisted increasingly of a mixture of drawing, digital photography, painting, written language, and externalized computer code, all of which were submitted to computational manipulations (including viral attacks)" (Nechvatal 2011). To produce his computer-robotic-assisted acrylics, Nechvatal worked with programmer Stephane Sikora, who created an artificial-life virus within the computer. The files are then transferred to a computer-driven robot, which paints with a brush onto canvas. He exhibited his work as prints, videos, and more complex robotic installations. The C++ custom virus program gradually invades, destroys, and transforms the artist's initial art images, literally recreating the artwork. Once launched, the artist is in no way able to predict how the virus will proceed to transform his work.

"On a planet that is increasingly technologically linked and globally mediated, how might noises break and re-connect in distinctive and productive ways within practices located in the world of art and thought?" Nechvatal asks (Nechvatal 2011). Using artificial-life viruses and the viral to study and demonstrate the viractual might provide an answer. In the books *Genesis* and *The Parasite,* Michel Serres defined the concept of noise as "the incident of interference" and as a parasite: "noise is a chaotic parasite that is an excluded middle (or third)—without which the entire logical structure of Western thought is unthinkable" (Nechvatal 2011, 16). Noise, in fact, "can block, distort, or change the meaning of a message in both human and electronic communication." Yet, the resulting interfered and transformed communication—that is, what is unacceptable because it corrupts an object or a phenomenon (both conceived as "pristine")—can suddenly become acceptable and even desirable when it transforms into something else. Nechvatal mentions the example of music: what was once considered noise has now turned into noise music, a genre in its own right.

Unlike those individuals and companies that have incorporated the viral into their own activities to attain enhanced productivity, Nechvatal refuses to exploit directly selected qualities of the viral to fit his own goals. Once he has launched his Artificial Life virus, he lets it act independent of any human intervention. In some installations, the observer can observe how the virus exercises its discretion in making its way across the digital canvas, transforming, modifying, and destroying the original images, following its own programmed logic. Letting the virus take over is both a demonstration of the work of the *viractual*, and a different, new approach to the viral. The virtual, impersonated by the progression of the virus, acts upon and merges with a pre-existent canvas designed by the artist, who then observes the virus reconfiguring the artwork and accepts it as a new one. Nechvatal does not attempt to direct the virus's movement to achieve particular aesthetic results or reach specific goals. He simply chooses the subjects of his artworks, knowing that the virus will act upon them.

Subjects that reveal the decay of the world, the body, or politics are favorites of the artist, as it is demonstrated by his *Computer Virus Project*, a series initiated in the early 1990s as a response to the HIV/AIDS pandemic. In it, the virus, acting as an analog of the HIV virus, transforms and degrades the image. "But here," Nechvatal explains, "the virus is also the basis of a creative process, producing newness in reference to the major influence of the virus on evolution in biological systems (Sikora, n.d.)." Michelle

A. Tavano describes his paintings as "ambiguously and androgynously sexually themed. As the computer virus continues to attack the image, its ambiguity becomes stronger" (Tavano 2011).

Several years after Nechvatal's *viractual* experiments, another non-interventionist approach—that is, an approach that refuses to appropriate the functions of viruses to produce controlled and predictable outcomes—made its debut at the 49th Venice Biennale's Slovenian Pavillion. A joint project of epidemiC and 0100101110101101.org, *Biennale.py* was the first virus ever exhibited inside an art institution. While the project promptly helped the art collective to gain abundant media attention (epidemiC 2002), this 2001 stunt cleverly appropriated the distributed behavioral features of viruses, as well as the entire apparatus of stereotypes associated with them. Launched on the opening day of the Biennale, the virus first appeared in printed form, as the script of code, written in Python, hanging on the wall of the Slovenian Pavilion; several other copies were printed on T-shirts and given to the audience. In the same way, a virus spreads from one host to others thanks to social interactions, the artistic virus was transmitted from the gallery to the outside world by the visitors themselves, who had become the hosts and the transmitters just after visiting the gallery.

Meanwhile, the real computer virus—the virus carrying the Python instructions, which were simultaneously printed and exhibited in the gallery and on the T-shirts carried by the audience—was released online. Although there now existed three versions of the virus, it was the explicit display of the code itself that attracted immediate attention and gathered a curious audience. The virus's code, normally invisible to those without specific knowledge of programming, was suddenly turned into a tangible, concrete object. The programming language used to write the virus contributed to its popularity. Python is a language that has a particular aesthetic appeal, because it can be constructed as a semi-coherent narrative by using variables and code syntax strategically (in this case, the text narrates the progression of a party, where the moment of infection is identified with actions evocative of sexual activity).

The project is certainly more than just a playful exercise. *Biennale.py* was, according to Luca Lampo, a member of epidemiC, an aesthetic experiment to demonstrate our capacity to create beauty using programming code. But what garnered immediate attention for the virus was not its aesthetics: the artists were likely fully aware that focusing on a virus's aesthetics rather than on its intrinsic and assumed characteristics as a potentially dangerous entity would not suffice to mitigate the virus's reputation. Here, the aesthetics' contribution not only created the material appearance of the virus, but also, and especially, revealed its ability to spread, in this case, to manifest in multiple forms and to be in different realms simultaneously. In addition, the strategies of display used in *Biennale.py* seem to confirm, not dispel, the suspicious nature of the virus. For instance, it is not a surprise that Symantec and Norton antivirus classified *Biennale.py* as a virus when it was released in the world. Yet, the authors insisted that the same virus was a work of art when it entered the gallery space, as if its threatening components were neutralized and its disruptive and transformative power ceased to exist. In other words, it was the clever use of the viral that contributed to the popularity of the artwork and its creators, and to their identification as a collective of artists with a subversive edge. It is true that the artists used code as an artistic medium. Once they had fabricated the virus, they played the unpredictable and distributed features of the viral to their advantage, without, however, attempting to manipulate them. They just let the virus do its—intimidating, suspicious, interdisciplinary, etc.—job.

The Viral Takes Charge, or, the Art of Taking Risks

The idea of engaging with the viral when the result of such an action is not only uncertain but also potentially dangerous is usually considered misguided and unfathomable. To a certain extent, radical choices involving, for instance, the use of experimental drugs or virotherapy on patients who literally had nothing to lose can be interpreted as either folly or extraordinary, depending on whether the results of the experiments were successful. Generally speaking, the decision to perform an untested experiment is deemed both irresponsible and the product of human hubris. However, it is also possible to view these experiments as forward-thinking—daring, fearless attempts to improve the life and health of patients by means of scientific discovery. Those who criticize these daring jumps into the void mention the myth of Prometheus and Dr. Frankenstein as cautionary tales of what happens when scientists and explorers reach too far. To be clear, the curse of Frankenstein, the story narrates, is not at all about reaching too far (or "playing God," as much popular media has wrongly posited), but about not taking responsibility for the achievement. Embracing the viral requires not only being risky, it also demands becoming aware of the potentials that lie ahead, and is about taking responsibility for what will unfold, whatever that is (Johnston 2018).

I am reminded here of the way that a number of self-proclaimed biohackers have reclaimed this ethos: in deciding to use biotechnologies to perform body modifications on themselves with the intention of enhancing or correcting their body, they take responsibility for their own decisions. But in these cases, responsibility is shown as an individual journey, with biohackers risking their own health and lives. Several biohackers, especially those who have surged to popularity thanks to spectacular stunts involving their own body, interpret this activity as a way to improve, heal, and modify their bodies. Biohackers employ, among other things, new, relatively inexpensive, and surprisingly precise gene-editing techniques, such as

CRISPR, new discoveries elevating the role of the microbiome and viral DNA as fundamental to our health, newly available technologies that can be manipulated, modified, and turned into futuristic prostheses, etc. (Kirksey 2020).

Responding to ethical concerns raised by media and institutional science about the implications of individuals with no formal science training, or no proper lab equipment performing unregulated and unmonitored modifications on themselves, biohackers responded that their activities only affect their own bodies, not other people's bodies. Their action is an act of self-determination, a way to take charge: "my body, my genes" (Pearlman 2017). This is certainly a good point, a reasonable defense of their acts of rebellion against a medical and a scientific system eager to subject individuals to hyperregulated and blackboxed procedures but unwilling to allow them to question such procedures and dismissing any independent pursuit of knowledge.

This is the case of Jo Zayner, a self-proclaimed biohacker and enthusiastic supporter of DIY science. Zayner rose to popularity when they sterilized their body in an attempt to perform a microbiome transplant to improve their digestion problems. Later on, they famously injected their arm publicly with DNA encoding for CRISPR that could theoretically enhance their muscles. Meant to demystify and promote bioengineering as a practice that could be learnt and accessed by everybody, Zayner's stunts inspired other people to take their body into their hands. Unfortunately, this led to risky experiments that could potentially endanger or even kill individuals whose health was already severely challenged by chronic conditions such as HIV/AIDS. In a later interview, Zayner said they regretted their stunts and called them "'social activism' gone awry" (Zhang 2018).

As interesting as the questioning of science and the act of taking charge expressed by most biohackers is, it must be acknowledged that it is often done in the name of self-improvement and self-enhancement (e.g., augmenting muscle mass, healing oneself of an annoying condition). Everybody is invited to participate in this self-hacking practice, but this practice rarely becomes a party. One of the main features of the viral is its ability to spread to more than one individual or a restricted group. It is a choral series of events. It is an infectious mechanism. Although biohacking generally claims to call for the involvement of a much larger crowd, it first calls upon the individual to make important decisions.

In 2012, Italian artist and activist Salvatore Iaconesi was diagnosed with glioblastoma, a complex form of brain cancer. He suddenly found himself in a situation, as he described it, where he felt that he was no longer a human being but had become "his own tumor." As doctors dispensed advice that felt to him orders to follow the typical standardized path of other patients with the same tumor, he found himself caught in a medical system intent on measuring, visualizing, and examining his condition only, one not seeing him as a whole person (Iaconesi 2013). In Iaconesi's words, "the patient is a strange being ... entirely made of data: blood exams, images of body parts, lab values, diagnoses" (Delfanti and Iaconesi 2016, 126). Not only did he realize that as a patient he was no longer considered an individual, but a fragmented entity, he also realized that even that resulting disembodied entity had been taken away from him. In fact, all the examinations that had been performed on him and that provided some important information on his condition as well as his body identity had been stored in a format impossible to share.

His reaction became *La Cura*, a long-term project that extends well beyond medical treatment or data sharing. Iaconesi rebelled against the reductive constraints imposed by medicine and sought to break free from an inflexible and impersonal medical system. He obtained and released his medical data online and turned to the community to seek advice, medical and otherwise. Here is where his endeavor acquired a much wider significance: his request, in fact, was not exclusively of a medical nature, but had a broader value, drawn by a need to open up "cancer's 'source code' as a biopolitical rite of healing, aimed at redefining concepts such as 'disease' and 'cure,'" " ... to re-appropriate the condition of being ill, and to foster a society that recognizes disease as a complex experience—one felt by social bodies as much as individual bodies" (124).

Iaconesi described his experience with the medical system as a ritual made of never-ending scans, repeated examinations, blood work, etc., during which both his body and his humanity were seen as fragments and as if they were simply a bundle of data: "your body, personality, and social connections disappear, and are replaced by data and images" (128). The use of the term *ritual* is telling: individuals performing a ritual are usually only partially aware of the meaning behind these actions. In fact, they are habitual, collective, and symbolic, performed as if to honor an authoritarian dogma whose meaning is not always evident but is respected nonetheless. Iaconesi was caught in a ritual where everything is obsessively quantified. His act of contravening the ritual subverted the system, turning him into a "bad patient"; he not only refused to abide by the "machinery of medicalization ritual," but also proceeded to share his data with unknown individuals.

For the medical field, the lesson to be learned from this extraordinary situation is that a similar interdisciplinary strategy may be useful to initiate a shift in the priorities of the medical field from data to affect and from quantification and purification to contextual and critical analysis. For the sake of our discussion on the viral, this story far exceeds issues of information gathering and dissemination, issues of disease and contagion, risk and control. Iaconesi was asked to explain what his intention was in becoming a "bad patient" and in reaching out to a wider community. What did he hope to achieve exactly? Was his goal to search for a better cure? This act of sharing was not meant to disseminate information with the purpose of receiving more. It was not meant to acquire knowledge to be used for his exclusive benefit. Iaconesi's act of sharing was projected outside, far away from his circle of intimate friends and trusted acquaintances; it was opened to a precarious and indeterminate space, just like the impatient seed in Kirstine Roepstorff's theatre piece introduced in the introduction opens to darkness and the unknown. By turning to a community made up of close friends and complete strangers, Iaconesi welcomed and eventually recovered human and affective elements that had been lost in the extreme operation of reduction he had endured during his experience in the medical system. His operation was a request to be infected and to infect, both materially and affectively. Materially, this request is meant to simultaneously receive, collect, and disseminate—practical, moral, emotional—advice and suggestions. Affectively, it is an attempt to reach out, to establish meaningful and human-dense contacts, to feel the pulse of a community and to create one.

This double gesture embodies the whole idea of the viral. It is also a gesture of care. Maria de la Bellacasa explains that caring is "everything that we do to maintain, continue and repair our world, so that we can live in it as well as possible" (Puig de la Bellacasa 2017, 3). Caring also means becoming aware that "studying and representing things have world-making effects" (30). It is a way of thinking and speaking beyond what we assume to be some social and "politically" useful research.

La Cura (the project led by Iaconesi and Oriana Persico) evolved to encompass workshops revolving around social issues, installations reflecting on more-than-human relationships between the human, the social, and the natural body, and has as one of its mottos, "the cure does not exist if not in society" (*La Cura* 2017). While critical of the objectification of the patient through a disproportionate faith in data, and of the cruelty that this faith can unleash when encapsulated in a bureaucratic system—the "horror of data," as he described the situation during a 2022 roundtable (ArtSci Salon 2022)—*La Cura* does not reject data. On the contrary, it uses data collection and data visualization in combination with social dialogue and meaningful sharing as if they were all part of a complex ecosystem. Data are only a part, not the protagonists, of the world. *La Cura* draws attention to the impossibility of understanding disease as a self-contained item or as a conglomerate of data. The important presence of the social and the emphasis on human relations underline the added value of the environmental and material conditions surrounding the body.

La Cura and its long-term performative journey into the meanderings of cancer research and management emphasize the role and use of affect in treating medical data (especially when it comes to personal medical data), and the necessity of regarding such data as part of a very complex (and therefore relational) context. Here, the visualization of medical data and cancer information, and other items used in diagnosing, curing, and, importantly, comforting the patient, become part of an affective ecology that combine different practices and link different individuals, fostering not only dialogues and discussions, but also artistic interventions and political considerations about care and social responsibility. Thus, becoming viral in this case is not at all about collecting bits and pieces of a puzzle that will draw a full picture, or that will help fully and completely comprehend the functioning of a disease (or a virus), a happy ending of sorts; it is not about reaching an established goal, but opening up to a new world and to chance; it is about embracing whatever unknown resolution will unfold. It is about embracing the viral and its unpredictable (but very logical) articulations.

8

Toward Viral Methodologies

In this book, I have offered a number of ways in which the viral circulates in digital and biological forms, as narratives, or as motifs and tropes spreading across literary texts, social media, and news media. Viruses and viral phenomena have been examined in their material nature and in their dynamic behavior by the biological sciences and computer sciences; their features have been purposely appropriated or adopted in creative ways and as ways of survival. Creative projects and alternative narratives have been used to address different aspects of viruses, their virological complexity, and entangled multiplicity, on the one hand, and their—metaphorical and material—epidemiological pervasiveness, on the other. The viral is the product of a number of articulations, forming an overarching category, denoting features that all viruses, or virus-derived entities appear to carry.

I have suggested that re-articulating these inscrutable entities using the notion of the viral may not fully help us decipher them, as their complex configuration and their entangled and relational nature complicate and compromise their comprehension. However, it can offer new ways to live with viral phenomena and other such occurrences; it could lead to the formulation of new methods to help break the over-structured delimitations of these phenomena into pre-defined categories and disciplinary siloes. Opening cross-disciplinary dialogues may facilitate the comprehension of viral phenomena and the viral and may foster new transversal knowledge.

In *The Three Ecologies*, Felix Guattari identifies three ecological registers: the environment (or natural), social relationships (the social), and subjectivities (the mental). "It is quite simply wrong," he wrote, "to regard action on the psyche, the socius, and the environment as separate" (Guattari 1989, 134). He proposed to "..question the whole of subjectivity and capitalist power formations—formations which, moreover, can by no means be assured of continuing the successes of the last decade" (Guattari 1989, 140). This new, transversal thinking rethinks categories and current norms through "effective practices of experimentation" that put these three ecologies in communication.

Disciplines, categories, and phenomena exist as the intersections of different and often non-compatible forces, such as those created by humans, their technologies and objects, instruments, and processes; the organic and the non-organic, images and their surrounding socio-cultural contexts. If examined from this angle, ecology becomes a powerful expression (Robbins 2004), taking in the whole spectrum of power dynamics that unfolds thanks to the friction and negotiation between its parts. This particular perspective helps capture how pre-constituted economies and the biosocial containment of artifacts and subjects take particular forms (as images or as instruments). By the same token, it may also reveal how these subjects and artifacts are configured, as Esposito observes, "to cope with or to construct certain events and assumptions" (Esposito 2008, 15).

These theoretical tenets become crucial in understanding viruses in ways that are not exclusionary or strictly disciplinary, but multifaceted. Given the intricacy of the web of relations that collect all viral manifestations under the same discourse, viruses cannot be studied as isolated entities that exist exclusively within distinct contexts. New strategies that examine viruses as substantial parts of this wider network of relations, intersections of forces, and exchanges have to be developed. Viruses neither exclusively affect our society, nor are they just being transformed and manipulated by technological devices or social-political agendas, but knowing that these possibilities exist may help formulate more sophisticated interpretations of the impact of viruses. It is equally complicated to distinguish the many layers of technological devices and software behind the images of the viruses we admire on journal covers. However, becoming aware that these layers and processes exist may lead to a more sober understanding of viruses.

Using a combination of approaches may help us become more aware of, and so better able to rethink, the existing tendency to view viruses in absolute terms, that is, as alien, as other. But the question that concerns me the most here is: would a transformation in the approach to viruses lead to, or conversely, be the product of a change in our perception of viruses? And could we extend this different perspective beyond viruses to, say, those phenomena that cannot fully be comprehended with our current tools? Would adopting this new approach change the way we fear or become anxious when thinking about them? In other words: how do we cope with the viral? I am reminded here of Bayo Akomolafe's essay about the coronavirus (Akomolafe 2020)

> If this is indeed a war, do we really want to win it? What if winning is the worst possible outcome we could imagine? Do we want to come out on top, stamp out this viral enemy, and restore agency to the cold ossified tentacles of the familiar? Are we sure this disruption is not what we want, what we've cried for in unvoiced ways? Should we not treat this opening as our grand *marronage*, our fugitive departure from exhausted cottonfields?

I am not sure an answer to all the above questions exists. It was late 2019 when I submitted the first draft of this book. In the past two years, I had to revise my content to reflect the changing situation and to reflect my own re-thinking of the viral. I remain firmly supporting the idea that it is indeed possible and even imperative to embrace the viral: this would mean becoming increasingly aware of the intricacies and the infinite connections that enable the viral, and the limitations of technoscience, alone, to tackle and neutralize it. It would mean learning how to acknowledge the uncertainty that pandemics, sudden security breaches and other cataclysms present to us. This acknowledgment cannot be taken lightly. I have become more aware of the impact that viral events can have on different individuals. It is easy to pontificate on the failure to grasp the complexity of the viral when its effects on individuals can be very severe. The pandemic has caused my position on viruses and on the viral to become more nuanced.

Despite the clear need for a different, overtly interdisciplinary, non-anthropocentric approach to research, the ability to statistically predict and anticipate events such as pandemics and malware attacks is crucial. Accepting viral uncertainty may feel daunting. Fear of viruses as potential, as unknown, and as tricksters, the anthropocentric tendency to try to contain, control, and manipulate the viral and its threats, and the continuing tendency to represent them as a self-contained other with disproportionate agency act to prevent the embracing of alternative interpretations.

Based on statistics and mathematical models, the tools at our disposal are good at quantifying, but terrible at interpreting the data collected in a context. I try to make sense of the many artistic expressions that have provided valuable reflections and shed new light on viruses and their socio-cultural impact. By illustrating different narratives, non-traditional methods of analysis and display, and by focusing on the affective qualities of viral pandemics and infectious diseases rather than on their quantified and quantifiable configuration, the artistic practices I have discussed provide interpretations of viruses, the viral, and viral networks that are substantially different from the ones we are accustomed to hearing.

However, if before the pandemic it was already difficult to think of facing uncertainty without speculating on possible outcomes, or take a leap of faith without worrying about catastrophic "what if" scenarios, today the pandemic seems to have limited or even shuttered all care-free and open ended futures. The pandemic brought in physical and emotional discomfort, as well as a lingering and diffused sense of uncertainty. While the arts have been crucial in articulating this discomfort and in imagining alternative scenarios, the question, "can we imagine unimaginable futures?" has now been substituted with: will we ever go back to our—apparently controllable—past lives?

This reaction is partially understandable: for most, the pandemic has brought profound instability and uncertainty, even though, to be fair, the world was already in a state of profound instability well before the pandemic;

we were already staring with complete powerlessness at the deepening of systemic inequalities and at a depleted social justice; the disintegration of a feeble social trust had been gradual and steady for many years. Still, the idea of "embracing the viral" in a postpandemic reality raises ethical and epistemological concerns: allegedly, I have become conflicted between a drive toward embracing the viral and an intense discomfort in practicing it. What really troubles me here is not caused by the pandemic at all. It is realizing, on the one hand, that thinking about uncertainty, precarity, and instability as something to be embraced is a very privileged mode of thinking. On the other hand, it is coming to terms with the fact that embracing the viral, embracing uncertainty is a much more courageous act than I had initially thought. Fascinated by viral phenomena and by the resilient behavior of a few individuals (mostly artists), I have been wondering whether the solution—or the mitigation—to the uncertainties brought about by the viral was to take it all in and learn how to coexist with it.

The fictional characters in Cárdenas and Mehrmand's *Virus.Circus* come to the realization that abiding by given security and protection rules is standing in the way of their quest for pleasure. They must embrace risk and the unknown if they want to obtain pleasure; they must trade security for uncertainty if they want to find out. Renouncing such gratification in favor of a secure yet pleasure-less life is a price they are not willing to pay. Their decision to indulge in pleasurable activities does not come from blind refusal to accept their situation, but from a conscious reflection that acknowledges the risks but chooses to act otherwise. Similarly, Whittaker's "infectious cycle" credits the tropes and iconic symbols that characterize outbreak narratives and the cycle of anxiety they cause by showcasing mainstream and popular reactions to outbreaks and infectious diseases, and simultaneously refusing to accept them as a given. Whittaker's body of work is emblematic of how the responses to infectious phenomena are as much collective as they are individual; they are profoundly diversified and situated (Figure 30). Virgil Ulam's merging with the virus/nanobot in *Blood Music* is neither violent nor painless: it is a transformation process that the protagonist decides to literally and materially embrace. Caitlin Berrigan's coexistence with, and befriending of, the virus that inhabited her body for a good part of her life produces a continuous dialogue, not a war. Salvatore Iaconesi and Oriana Persico's *La Cura* extends well beyond finding a cure for a deadly condition: it is a way to reach for and create a rich and harmonious community where care, not competition; long-lasting solidarity, not immediate outcomes; and community data, not data colonization are at the core.

It is curiosity, rather than fear, that captures the impatient seed protagonist of Kirstine Roepstorff's *Influenza, Theatre of Glowing Darkness* mentioned at the beginning of this book. In this case, the anxious not-knowing of the seed is transformed into anticipation and excitement to be savored and even enjoyed before light breaks in. When I visited the Biennale and came across Roepstorff's immersive installation, I found myself rooting for the seed, its

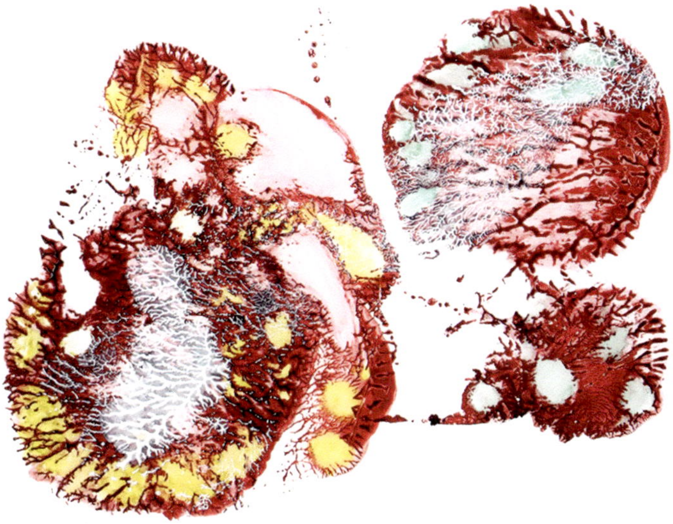

FIGURE 30 *Elaine Whittaker,* Pandemic Convergence, *2020. Acrylic on Paper. © Elaine Whittaker.*

impatience, and its youthful spirit of adventure. It was maybe because I have always had a sweet spot for the brave and the mad risk taker, the rebel and the misfit, or maybe because my experience of the piece, with its intense sensory stimulations, and its appeal to the spectator's curiosity led me to. In fact, the piece was designed to evoke a sense of impatience: it started from the lineup to access the limited capacity show, and continued inside the sweltering room, when the spectators were sat on tall chairs in complete darkness.

But that was 2017.
Is it still possible to root for the seed?

During a performance/video titled "*staying in touch: post-coronavirus art curating*" five artists converging in the virtual residency "Braiding Fiction" developed a speculative fiction in which art is the virus and art practitioners act as front-line workers. The result is a fictional interview with the curators offering a series of important reflections on the future of art, human proximity, and coexisting with the viral. "I would rather die than live in a world where art spaces are closed," exclaims AN (Anise Neuchâtel), one of the curators of a fictional exhibition (Mackenzie et al. 2021). Her expression contains a subtle criticism of the rush toward going exclusively virtual by most galleries and museums during the coronavirus pandemic. "There is no old normal." " ... there is no normal." While we must continue to live, work, and exhibit art, attempting to return to a pre-pandemic order is unlikely, if not impossible. Therefore, it is important to continue to find new ways of coexistence. Another fictional curator, VL (Vess L) explains that the idea of art as an isolated object may be outdated in a post-pandemic era: "art not only becomes a part of the workplace, it becomes a part of the home, it becomes a part of the infrastructure of a city, it becomes part of the environment in an all-encompassing and really comprehensive way." Art may go viral after all.

References

Acheson, N. H. (2011), *Fundamentals of Molecular Virology*, 2nd ed., Hoboken, NJ: John Wiley & Sons.
Adam, D. (2020), "Special Report: The Simulations Driving the World's Response to COVID-19", *Nature*, 580 (7803): 316–18.
Adams, D. (1995), *The Hitchhiker's Guide to the Galaxy*, New York: Del Rey.
Ahmed, S. (2010), *The Promise of Happiness*, Durham, NC: Duke University Press.
Aickelin, U. and S. Cayzer (2002), "The Danger Theory and Its Application to Artificial Immune Systems", Available at SSRN: https://ssrn.com/abstract=2832054 or http://dx.doi.org/10.2139/ssrn.2832054 (accessed January 1, 2002).
Akomolafe, B. (2020), "I, Coronavirus. Mother. Monster. Activist", *Emergence Network* (blog), Available online http://www.emergencenetwork.org/icoronavirus/ (accessed on April 13, 2020).
Alt, C. (2005), "Viral Load. The Fantastic Rhetorical Power of the Computer Virus in the Post-9/11 Political Landscape", *OZG—Oesterreichisce Zeitschrift Für Geschitswissenshaften*, 3 (16): 133–49.
Andersen, K. G., A. Rambaut, W. I. Lipkin, E. C. Holmes and R. F. Garry (2020), "The Proximal Origin of SARS-CoV-2", *Nature Medicine*, 26 (4): 450–2.
ArtSci Salon (2022), "Beyond Triage and Data Culture", *Who Cares? Sustaining Relations of Health beyond the Time of Crisis*. https://artscisalon.com/who-cares/.
ArtTheScience (2018), "Features—Screened for by Elaine Whittaker", *Polyfield Magazine*, Available online https://artthescience.com/magazine/2018/03/20/features-screened-for/ (accessed December 28, 2021).
Ashley, J., B. Cordy, D. Lucia, L. G. Fradkin, V. Budnik and T. Thomson (2018), "Retrovirus-like Gag Protein Arc1 Binds RNA and Traffics across Synaptic Boutons", *Cell*, 172 (1–2): 262–74. e11.
Axelsson, S. and D. Sands (2006), *Understanding Intrusion Detection through Visualization*, vol. 24, New York: Springer.
Aycock, J. (2006), *Computer Viruses and Malware*, vol. 22, New York: Springer.
Aycock, J. and A. Maurushat (2008), "'Good' Worms and Human Rights", *ACM SIGCAS Computers and Society*, 38 (1): 28–39. https://doi.org/10.1145/1361255.1361256.
Bak, A. and J. B. Emerson (2020), "Cauliflower Mosaic Virus (CaMV) Biology, Management, and Relevance to GM Plant Detection for Sustainable Organic Agriculture", *Frontiers in Sustainable Food Systems*, 4: 21.
Ball, P. and A. Maxmen (2020). "The Epic Battle against Coronavirus Misinformation and Conspiracy Theories", *Nature*, 581 (7809): 371–4.
Baluska, F. (2009), "Cell-Cell Channels, Viruses, and Evolution: Via Infection, Parasitism, and Symbiosis toward Higher Levels of Biological Complexity", *Annals of the New York Academy of Sciences*, 1178: 106–19.

Barabási, A.-L. (2003), *Linked: How Everything Is Connected to Everything Else and What It Means for Business, Science, and Everyday Life*, New York: Plume.
Barad, K. (2007), *Meeting the Universe Halfway: Quantum Physics and the Entanglement of Matter and Meaning*, Durham: Duke University Press.
Barad, K. (2014), "Invertebrate Visions: Diffractions of the Brittlestar", in E. Kirksey (ed), *The Multispecies Salon*, 221–41, Durham: Duke University Press.
Barber, C. (2020), "The Problem of 'Long Haul' COVID", *Scientific American*, Available online https://www.scientificamerican.com/article/the-problem-of-long-haul-covid/ (accessed on December 29, 2020).
Bardini, T. (2016), "Future Life Will Be Synthetic: About the Emergence of Engineered Life, Its Promises, Prophecies and the Formal Causalities Needed to Make Sense of Them", *Social Science Information*, 55 (3): 369–84.
Barnes, D. (2020), *60-Second Lectures in Quarantine: "Surviving Plagues Past and Present"*, Available online https://vimeo.com/414990534.
Baudrillard, J. (1995), *The Gulf War Did Not Take Place*, Bloomington: Indiana University Press.
Bauman, Z. (2005), *Liquid Life*, Cambridge, MA: Polity Press.
Bauman, Z. (2006), *Liquid Fear*, Cambridge, MA: Polity Press.
BBC News (2020), "DR Congo's Deadliest Ebola Outbreak Declared Over", Available online https://www.bbc.com/news/world-africa-53179323 (accessed on June 25, 2020).
Bear, G. (1983), "Blood Music", *Analog Magazine*.
Bear, G. (1986), *Blood Music*, New York: Ace Books.
Bell, J. C., K. A. Garson, B. D. Lichty and D. F. Stojdl (2002). "Oncolytic Viruses: Programmable Tumour Hunters", *Current Gene Therapy*, 2 (2): 243–54.
Bennett, J. (2010), *Vibrant Matter: A Political Ecology of Things*, Durham: Duke University Press.
la Berge, A. E. Fowler (1999), "The History of Science and the History of Microscopy", *Perspectives on Science*, 7 (1): 111–42.
Berlin, J. (2020), "Know That Coronavirus Image with Red Spikes? Here's How the Artists at the CDC Created It", *Chicago Tribune*, April 4, 2020, online edition, sec. Coronavirus, Available online https://www.chicagotribune.com/coronavirus/ct-viz-coronavirus-how-it-was-drawn-20200403-ka4t4zyab5ejpcp5y7ukn2mb4u-story.html.
Berrigan, C. (2009), "Life Cycle of a Common Weed", MFA Diss, Massachusetts Institute of Technologies.
Berrigan, C. (2012), "The Life Cycle of a Common Weed: Reciprocity, Anxiety, and the Aesthetic of Noncatharsis", *Women's Studies Quarterly*, 40 (1 & 2): 97–116.
Berrigan, C. (2020), "Atmospheres of the Undead: Living with Viruses, Loneliness, and Neoliberalism", *MARCH. A Journal of Art and Strategy*, Available online https://march.international/atmospheres-of-the-undead-living-with-viruses-loneliness-and-neoliberalism/ (accessed in September 2020).
Blas, Z. (2012), "Viral", *Women's Studies Quarterly*, 40 (1 & 2): 29–39.
Blystad, D.-R. (2020), "Viral Life Symposium", November 17, 2020, Available online https://virallife.vitenparken.no/symposium/.
Boase, J. and B. Wellman (2001), "A Plague of Viruses: Biological, Computer and Marketing", *Current Sociology*, 49 (6): 39–55.

Bontchev, V. (1994), "Are 'Good' Computer Viruses Still a Bad Idea?", Virus Test Center, Hamburg, Available online https://bontchev.nlcv.bas.bg/papers/goodvir.html (accessed in September 2009).

Boot, M. (2020), "The Three Reasons Conspiracy Theories Are More Dangerous than Ever", *Washington Post*, Available online https://www.washingtonpost.com/opinions/2020/05/23/three-reasons-conspiracy-theories-are-more-dangerous-than-ever/ (accessed on May 23, 2020).

Bos, L. (1999), "The Naming of Viruses: An Urgent Call to Order", *Archives of Virology*, 144 (3): 631–6.

Bos, L. (2000), "100 Years of Virology: From Vitalism via Molecular Biology to Genetic Engineering", *Trends in Microbiology*, 8 (2): 82–7.

Boustead, G. (2009), "At the Edge of Perception. Luke Jerram's Work Explores the Limits of Science and Art, Challenging the Boundaries of Both", *Seed Magazine*, October 15, 2009.

Bowls, S. (2014), "'Blair Witch Project': Still a Legend 15 Years Later", *USA TODAY*, Available online https://www.usatoday.com/story/life/movies/2014/07/13/blair-witch-project-15th-anniversary-classic-legend/10707409/ (accessed on July 13, 2014).

Box, G. E. P. (1976), "Science and Statistics", *Journal of the American Statistical Association*, 71 (356): 791–9.

boyd, D. and K. Crawford (2012), "Critical Questions for Big Data", *Information, Communication & Society*, 15 (5): 662–79. https://doi.org/10.1080/1369118X.2012.678878.

Brives, C. (2021), "Pluribiosis and the Never-Ending Microgeohistories", in M. R. S. Sariola and C. Brives (eds), *With Microbes*, 247–67, Mattering Press.

Brockman, D. (2007), "Auf den Spuren des Geldes - Neue Wege fur Modelle zur geographischen Seuchenausbreitung", Research Yearbook, Max Planck Institut Fur Dynamik und Selbstorganisation.

Brossard, D. and B. V. Lewenstein (2010), "A Critical Appraisal of Models of Public Understanding of Science", in L. Kahlor and P. Stout (eds), *Communicating Science. New Agendas in Communication*, 11–17, New York: Routledge.

Buchen-Osmond, C. (2003), "Taxonomy and Classification of Viruses", in P. R. Murray and E. J. Baron (eds), *Manual of Clinical Microbiology*, 1217–26, Washington, DC: ASM Press.

Buiani, R. (2009), "Viral Games in the Networked World", in J. Parikka and T. Sampson (eds), The Spam Book. On Spam, Porn and Other Anomalous Objects in Digital Culture, 81–100, Cresskill, NJ: Hampton Press.

Buiani, R. (2014), "Innovation and Compliance in Making and Perceiving the Scientific Visualization of Viruses", *Canadian Journal of Communication*, 39 (4): 539–57.

Buiani, R. (2021), "All Models Are Wrong, but Some Are Useful: Mathematical Models at the Time of COVID 19", *Punctum. International Journal of Semiotics*, 7 (1): 115–30.

Burgess, J. (2012), "The iPhone Moment, the Apple Brand, and the Creative Consumer: From 'Hackability and Usability' to Cultural Generativity", in L. Hjorth, J. Burgess and I. Richardson (eds), *Studying Mobile Media: Cultural Technologies, Mobile Communication, and the iPhone*, 35–50, New York: Routledge.

Cairo, A. (2016), *The Truthful Art: Data, Charts, and Maps for Communication*, San Francisco: New Riders.

Callier, V. (2018), "Interspecies Hybrids Play a Vital Role in Evolution", *Quanta Magazine*.

Campbell-Dollaghan, K. (2014), "Here's an Illustrated Guide to the World's Worst Computer Viruses", *Gizmodo*. Available online: https://gizmodo.com.au/2014/07/heres-an-illustrated-guide-to-the-worlds-worst-computer-viruses/.

Cann, A. J. (2012), *Principles of Molecular Virology*, 5th ed., Amsterdam: Elsevier; Waltham, MA: Academic Press.

Card, S. K., J. Mackinlay and B. Shneiderman, eds (1999), *Readings in Information Visualization: Using Vision to Think*, 1st edition, San Francisco, CA: Morgan Kaufmann.

Cárdenas, M., Z. Blas and W. Schirmacher (2011), *The Transreal: Political Aesthetics of Crossing Realities*, eds. Z. Blas and W. Schirmacher, New York, Atropos press.

Carrera, E. and G. Erdélyi (2004), "Digital Genome Mapping: Advanced Binary Malware Analysis", *Proceedings of the 14th Virus Bulletin Conference*, 187–97.

Cartwright, L. (1995), *Screening the Body: Tracing Medicine's Visual Culture*, Minneapolis: University of Minnesota Press.

Casini, S. (2010), "The Aesthetics of Magnetic Resonance Imaging (MRI): From the Scientific Laboratory to an Artwork", *Contemporary Aesthetics*, 8.

Caulfield, T. (2020), "The COVID-19 'Infodemic'—Debunking Works, If It's Done Right", *thestar.com*, June 19.

Cazeaux, C. (2015), "The Aesthetics of the Scientific Image", *Journal of Aesthetics and Phenomenology*, 2 (2): 187–209.

CBC News (2021), "Ontario Issues Stay-at-Home Order as COVID-19 Models Show Province Is at 'dangerous Point' | CBC News", *CBC*, Available online: https://www.cbc.ca/news/canada/toronto/ontario-covid-modelling-jan-12-1.5868797 (accessed June 11, 2021).

CDC (2020), "Details—Public Health Image Library (PHIL)", Available online: https://phil.cdc.gov/Details.aspx?pid=23311 (accessed October 30, 2020).

Cepelewicz, J. (2017), "Interspecies Hybrids Play a Vital Role in Evolution", *Quanta Magazine*.

Cepelewicz, J. (2021), "The Hard Lessons of Modeling the Coronavirus Pandemic", *Quanta Magazine*, January 28.

Cetina, K. K. (1999), *Epistemic Cultures: How the Sciences Make Knowledge*, 1st edition, Cambridge, MA: Harvard University Press.

Chan, M. (2006), "Pandemic Flu—Communicating the Risks", *Bulletin of the World Health Organization*, 84 (1): 9–10.

Chandler, D. E. and R. W. Roberson (2009), *Bioimaging: Current Concepts in Light and Electron Microscopy*, Sudbury, MA: Jones and Bartlett Publishers.

Chang, K. (2020), "A University Had a Great Coronavirus Plan, but Students Partied On", *The New York Times*, September 10.

Chatterjee, S. (2020), "Visualizing the Virus", Available at https://visualizingthevirus.com/.

Chatterjee, S. (2020b), "Making the Invisible Visible: How We Depict COVID-19", *LSE School of Social Policy Blog*, Available online: https://blogs.lse.ac.uk/covid19/2020/06/30/making-the-invisible-visible-how-we-depict-covid-19/.

Chatterjee, S., A. Roy, A. Laskar and S. Swarnakar (2013), "Electron Microscopy in the Perspective of Modern Biology: Ultravision and Ultradimension", in A. Méndez-Vilas (ed), *Current Microscopy Contributions to Advances in Science and Technology*, 891–902, Badajoz: Formatex Research Center.

Chen, A. (2017), "How to Create a New Life Form: Historian Sophia Roosth on the Future of Synthetic Biology—The Verge", *The Verge*.
Chen, C. (1999), *Information Visualisation and Virtual Environments*, London; New York: Springer.
Chen, C. (2003), *Mapping Scientific Frontiers: The Quest for Knowledge Visualization*, London; New York: Springer.
Chen, C. (2004), *Information Visualization: Beyond the Horizon*, New York: Springer.
Chen, C. (2005), "Top 10 Unsolved Information Visualization Problems", *IEEE Computer Graphics and Applications*, 25 (4): 12–16.
Chen, C. (2019), *Victorian Contagion: Risk and Social Control in the Victorian Literary Imagination*, New York: Routledge.
Cheong, I. R. and M. R. Kidd (1997), "Safe Practices in Cyberspace: A Medical Perspective on Computer Viruses", *MJA*, 166 (44): 44–6.
Christiansen, J., M. Fischetti, V. Falconieri Hays and B. Glaunsinger (2020), "A Visual Guide to the SARS-CoV-2 Coronavirus", *Scientific American Newsletter*, Available online: https://www.scientificamerican.com/article/a-visual-guide-to-the-sars-cov-2-coronavirus/.
Clough, P. and J. Puar (2012), "Viral | The Feminist Press", *Women's Studies Quarterly*, 40 (1 & 2): 13–26.
Clough, P. T. (2008), "The Affective Turn: Political Economy, Biomedia and Bodies", *Theory, Culture & Society*, 25 (1): 1–22.
Cobián Güemes, A. G., M. Youle, V. A. Cantú, B. Felts, J. Nulton and F. Rohwer (2016), "Viruses as Winners in the Game of Life", *Annual Review of Virology*, 3 (1): 197–214.
Cohen, E. (2011), "The Paradoxical Politics of Viral Containment; or, How Scale Undoes Us One and All", *Social Text*, 29 (1 [106]): 15–35.
Cohen, F. (1987), "Computer Viruses: Theory and Experiments", *Computers and Security*, 6 (1): 22–35.
Cohen, F. (1991), "Current Best Practice against Computer Viruses", in *Proceedings. 25th Annual 1991 IEEE International Carnahan Conference on Security Technology*, 261–70, Taipei, Taiwan.
Cohen, F. B. (1992), "A Case for Benevolent Viruses" *DPMA, IEEE, ACM Computer Virus and Security Conference*, March 1992.
Cohen, F. B. (1994), *A Short Course on Computer Viruses*, New York; Toronto: Wiley.
Cohen, F. B. (1995), *Protection and Security on the Information Highway*, New York: John Wiley & Sons.
Contagion (2011), [Film], Dir. Steven Soderbergh, USA Warner Bros.
Coopmans, C. (2014), "Visual Analytics as Artful Revelation", in J. Vertesi, M. E. Lynch, S. Woolgar and C. Coopmans (eds), *Representation in Scientific Practice Revisited*, 37–60, Cambridge, MA: The MIT Press.
Coronavirus resource center (2020), "COVID-19 Map FAQ", *Johns Hopkins Coronavirus Resource Center*, Available online: https://coronavirus.jhu.edu/map-faq (accessed 14 July 2020).
Corum, J. and C. Zimmer (2020), "Bad News Wrapped in Protein: Inside the Coronavirus Genome", *The New York Times*, April 3.
Corum, J., D. Grady, S.-L. Wee and C. Zimmer (2020), "Coronavirus Vaccine Tracker", *The New York Times*.

Cosslett, V. E. (1951), *Practical Electron Microscopy*, London: Butterworths Scientific Publications.
Coy, P. (1996), "Andersen Consulting: Data Visualization: The Final Frontier?", *Bloomberg.com*, 28 October, Available online: https://www.bloomberg.com/news/articles/1996-10-28/andersen-consulting-data-visualization-the-final-frontier.
Crawford, D. H. (2000), *The Invisible Enemy: A Natural History of Viruses*, Oxford: Oxford University Press.
Cressey, D. and E. Callaway (2017), "Cryo-Electron Microscopy Wins Chemistry Nobel", *Nature News*, 550 (7675): 167.
Critical Art Ensemble (2006), *Marching Plague: Germ Warfare and Global Public Health*, Brooklyn, NY: Autonomedia.
Critical Art Ensemble (2008), "Tactical Media at Dusk?", *Third Text*, 22 (5): 535–48.
Cuthand, R. (n.d.), "Trading Series", *Ruth Cuthand*.
Dalton, C. and J. Thatcher (n.d.), "What Does a Critical Data Studies Look like, and Why Do We Care? Seven Points for a Critical Approach to 'Big Data'", *Environment and Planning D: Society and space*, Big Data Critical Data Studies.
Dalton, C. M., L. Taylor and J. Thatcher (alphabetical) (2016), "Critical Data Studies: A Dialog on Data and Space", *Big Data & Society*, 3 (1): 2053951716648346.
Danon, L., A. P. Ford, T. House, C. P. Jewell, M. J. Keeling, G. O. Roberts, J. V. Ross, M. C. Vernon (2011), "Networks and the Epidemiology of Infectious Disease", *Interdisciplinary Perspectives on Infectious Diseases*, 2011: e284909.
Dasgupta, D., S. Yu and F. Nino (2011), "Recent Advances in Artificial Immune Systems: Models and Applications", *Applied Soft Computing*, The Impact of Soft Computing for the Progress of Artificial Intelligence, 11 (2): 1574–87.
Daston, L. and P. Galison (1992), "The Image of Objectivity", *Representations*, (40): 81–128.
Daston, L. J. and P. Galison (2010), *Objectivity*, Cambridge, MA: The MIT Press.
Davis, M., P. Flowers, D. Lohm, E. Waller and N. Stephenson (2016), "Immunity, Biopolitics and Pandemics: Public and Individual Responses to the Threat to Life", *Body & Society*, 22 (4): 130–54.
Davis, N. (2017), "What Is Cryo-Electron Microscopy, the Nobel Prize-Winning Technique?" *The Guardian*, October 4.
Dayrat, B. (2005), "Towards Integrative Taxonomy", *Biological Journal of the Linnean Society*, 85 (3): 407–15.
de Lange, C. (2014), "Print a Virus to Kill the Cancer", *New Scientist*, 224 (2999): 28–9.
Deleuze, G. (2006), *Foucault*, London: Continuum International Publishing Group.
Delfanti, A. and S. Iaconesi (2016), "Open Source Cancer. Brain Scans and the Rituality of Biodigital Data Sharing", in D. Barney, G. Coleman, C. Ross, J. Sterne and T. Tembek (eds), *The Participatory Condition in the Digital Age*, 123–44, Minneapolis, MN: University of Minnesota Press.
de Sousa Santos, B. (2020), "Virus: All That Is Solid Melts into Air", *Blog of the APA*.
Devlin, H. and N. Davis (2017), "Nobel Prize in Chemistry Awarded for Method to Visualise Biomolecules", *The Guardian*, October 4.

Dewdney, A. K. (1984), "In the Game Called 'CORE War' Hostile Programs Engage in a Battle of Bits", *Scientific American*, 5 (250): 14.
Dewdney, A. K. (1985), "A Core War Bestiary of Viruses, Worms and Other Threats to Computer Memories", *Scientific American*, 3 (250) (March): 14.
Dewdney, A. K. (1989), "Of Worms, Viruses and Core War", *Scientific American*, 260 (3): 90–3.
D'Ignazio, C. and L. F. Klein (2020), *Data Feminism*, Cambridge, MA: MIT Press.
Dibbell, J. (1995), "Viruses Are Good for You", *Wired Magazine* (February).
Dimka, J. L. (2015), "Modeling the Spread of the 1918 Influenza Pandemic in a Newfoundland Community", Thesis, University of Missouri–Columbia.
Dimmock, J., A. J. Easton and K. N. Leppard (2001), *Introduction to Modern Virology*, Oxford: Blackwell Science.
Dols, M. W. (1974), "Plague in Early Islamic History", *Journal of the American Oriental Society*, 94 (3): 371–83.
Dominguez, R. (2020), "Infodemics: Going Viral, or Undead Media", *Contactos*.
Dong, E., H. Du and L. Gardner (2020), "An Interactive Web-Based Dashboard to Track COVID-19 in Real Time", *The Lancet Infectious Diseases*, 20 (5): 533–4.
Draculescu, A. (n.d.), "Alex Dragulescu—Works Catalog", Available online: http://www.sq.ro/ (accessed November 25, 2012).
Dreifus, C. (1998), "A Conversation with Polly Matzinger; Blazing an Unconventional Trail to a New Theory of Immunity", *The New York Times*, June 16.
Dror, O. Y. (1999), "The Scientific Image of Emotion: Experience and Technologies of Inscription", *Configurations*, 7 (3): 355–401.
Dror, O. Y. (2001), "Counting the Affects: Discoursing in Numbers", *Social Research*, 68 (2): 357–78.
Dubochet, J. (2012), "Cryo-EM—the First Thirty Years", *Journal of Microscopy*, 245 (3): 221–4.
Duff, T. (2009), "Going Viral: Live Performance and Documentation in the Science Laboratory", *Performance Research*, 14 (4): 36–44.
Duff, T. (2011), "Living Viral Tattoos? Crisis Alert!" *TOTAL ART*, 1 (1): 1–9.
Duff, T. (2012), "Cryobook Archives", *Canadian Journal of Communication*, 37 (1): 147–54.
Duff, T., J. Muhling, M. G. Godinho and S. Hodgetts (2011), "How to Make Living Viral Tattoos", *Leonardo*, 44 (2): 164–5.
Duhaime-Ross, Arielle (2014), "Ebola Panic Is Getting Pretty Racist", *The Verge*.
Dumitriu, A. (2021), "Ex Voto", *Anna Dumitriu* (blog). https://annadumitriu.co.uk/portfolio/ex-voto/ (accessed August 16, 2021).
Dupré, J. and S. Guttinger (2016), "Viruses as Living Processes", *Studies in History and Philosophy of Science Part C: Studies in History and Philosophy of Biological and Biomedical Sciences*, 59: 109–16.
Earl, L. A., V. Falconieri, J. L. Milne and S. Subramaniam (2017), "Cryo-EM: Beyond the Microscope", *Current Opinion in Structural Biology, Cryo Electron Microscopy: Exciting Advances in CryoEM Herald a New Era in Structural Biology. Biophysical Methods: Behind the Scenes of the Cryo-EM Revolution*, 46: 71–8.
'Ebola: Mapping the Outbreak' (2016), *BBC News*, January 14.
Epidemic (2002), "Brand Virus", *Bocconi News*: *http://www.uni-bocconi.it* (May 6th).
Epstein, M. A. (2001), "Historical Background", *Philosophical transactions of the Royal Society of London-Series B: Biological Sciences* (356): 413–20 (2011).

Epstein, S. (1996), *Impure Science: AIDS, Activism, and the Politics of Knowledge*, 1st edition, Berkeley, CA: University of California Press.
Ero (2004), *Graphing Malware*, F-Secure Website, Available online: https://archive.f-secure.com/weblog/archives/00000324.
Esposito, R. (2008), *Bíos: Biopolitics and Philosophy*, Minneapolis: University of Minnesota Press.
Ewald, P. W. (2004), "Evolution of Virulence", *Infectious Disease Clinics of North America*, 18 (1): 1–15.
F-Secure (2007), *FS-CSI*. Available online at https://archive.f-secure.com/weblog/archives/00001225.
F-secure (2008), *Weblog*, F-secure website, Available online: https://archive.f-secure.com/weblog/archives/.
Falconieri Hays, V. (2020), "How I Built a 3-D Model of the Coronavirus for Scientific American", *Scientific American*, June 25, Available online: https://www.scientificamerican.com/article/how-i-built-a-3-d-model-of-the-coronavirus-for-scientific-american/.
Faria, N. R., et al. (2016), "Zika Virus in the Americas: Early Epidemiological and Genetic Findings", *Science*, 352 (6283): 345–9.
Ferguson, N., D. Laydon, G. Nedjati Gilani, et al. (2020), "Report 9: Impact of Non-Pharmaceutical Interventions (NPIs) to Reduce COVID19 Mortality and Healthcare Demand", Report. https://doi.org/10.25561/77482.
Fernandes, D. A. B., M. M. Freire, P. A. P. Fazendeiro and P. R. M. Inácio (2017), "Applications of Artificial Immune Systems to Computer Security: A Survey", *Journal of Information Security and Applications*, 35: 138–59.
Fine, P., C. G. Victora, K. J. Rothman, P. S. Moore, Y. Chang, V. Curtis, D. L. Heymann, G. Slutkin, R. M. May, V. Patel, I. Roberts, R. Wortley, C. Torgerson and A. Deaton (2013), "John Snow's Legacy: Epidemiology without Borders", *Lancet*, 381 (9874): 1302–11.
Fishel, S. R. (2017), *The Microbial State: Global Thriving and the Body Politic*, Minneapolis: University of Minnesota Press.
Flegler, S. L., J. W. Heckman and K. L. Klomparens (1993), *Scanning and Transmission Electron Microscopy: An Introduction*, New York: W.H. Freeman.
Flegler, S. L., J. W. Heckman Jr and K. L. Klomparens (1997), *Scanning and Transmission Electron Microscopy: An Introduction*, New Ed., USA: Oxford University Press.
Fontenelle, B. L. B. de, H. A. Hargreaves, and N. R. Gelbart (2000), *Conversations on the Plurality of Worlds*, Nachdr., Berkeley, CA: University of California Press.
Forrest, S. and A. Somayaji (1997), "Computer Immunology", *Communication of the ACM*, 40 (10): 88–97.
Forrest, S. and C. Beauchemin (2007), "Computer Immunology, Department of Computer Science, University of New Mexico", *Immunological reviews*, 216 (1): 176–97.
Forrest, S. and S. Hofmayer (2000), "Architecture for an Artificial Immune System", *Evolutionary computational journal*, 8 (4): 443–73.
Forterre, P. and D. Prangishvili (2009), "The Origin of Viruses", *Research in Microbiology*, 160 (7): 466–72.
Foucault, M. (1981), *Power/Knowledge: Selected Interviews and Other Writings*, New York: Panthenon Books.

Foucault, M. (1989a), *The Archaeology of Knowledge*, London; New York: Routledge.
Foucault, M. (1989b), *The Order of Things*, London; New York: Routledge.
Foucault, M. (1994), *The Birth of the Clinic: An Archaeology of Medical Perception*, New York: Vintage.
Foucault, M. (2003), *Society Must Be Defended: Lectures at the Collège de France, 1975–76*, eds, M. Bertani, A. Fontana, F. Ewald and D. Macey, New York: Picador.
Foucault, M. (2007), *Security, Territory, Population: Lectures at the Collège de France, 1977–1978*, eds, M. Senellart and A. I. Davidson, Basingstoke: Palgrave Macmillan.
Foucault, M. (2008), *The Birth of Biopolitics: Lectures at the Collège de France, 1978–79*, eds, M. Senellart and C. de France, Basingstoke England; New York: Palgrave Macmillan.
Frattini, G. O. (2021), "Laura Splan's Entangled Entities, Intertwining Art & Biotech," *CLOT Magazine*.
Friendly, M. (2008), "A Brief History of Data Visualization", *Handbook of Data Visualization*, Springer Handbooks Comp. Statistics, 15–56, Berlin: Springer.
Frost, N. (2020), "Quarantined for Life: The Tragic History of US Leprosy Colonies", *HISTORY*, Available online: https://www.history.com/news/leprosy-colonies-us-quarantine (accessed August 17, 2021).
Frow, E. (2014), "In Images We Trust? Representation and Objectivity in the Digital Age", in C. Coopmans, J. Vertesi, M. E. Lynch and S. Woolgar (eds), *Representation in Scientific Practice Revisited*, 249–68, Cambridge, MA: The MIT Press.
Frumkin, R. (2020), "How to Draw the Coronavirus", *The Paris Review*.
Fry, H. (2021), "When Graphs Are a Matter of Life and Death | The New Yorker", *The New Yorker*.
Gaiter, C. (2020), "Visualizing the Virus", *The Conversation*. Available online at http://theconversation.com/visualizing-the-virus-135415.
Gallery 400 (2021), "Biological Agents—Gallery 400", October 12–November 22 2008.
Galloway, A. R. and E. Thacker (2007), *The Exploit: A Theory of Networks*, Minneapolis: University of Minnesota Press.
Gelderblom, H. R. (1996), "Structure and Classification of Viruses", 4th edn, in S. Baron (ed), *Medical Microbiology*, Galveston, TX: University of Texas Medical Branch at Galveston, Available onliine: https://www.ncbi.nlm.nih.gov/books/NBK8174/.
Generation Like (2014), [TV program] PBS Frontline, August 5
Genosko, G. (2006), "The Case of Mafiaboy and the Rhetorical Limits of Hacktivism", *Fibreculture* (9), Available online: https://nine.fibreculturejournal.org/fcj-057/.
gergo (2005), *A Different Look at Bagle*, F-Secure webpost archive, Available online: https://archive.f-secure.com/weblog/archives/00000662.
Gerlach, N. and S. N. Hamilton (2014), "Trafficking in the Zombie: The CDC Zombie Apocalypse Campaign, Diseasseability and Pandemic Culture", *Refractory* (June 26).
Ghosh, A. (2016), *The Great Derangement: Climate Change and the Unthinkable*, Chicago: University Of Chicago Press.

Giaimo, C. (2020), “The Spiky Blob Seen around the World”, *The New York Times*, April 1.
GISP and E. Geraghty (2020), “Mapping Epidemics: From SARS, Zika, and Ebola to the Pandemic of COVID-19”, *Esri*.
Goldsmith, C. S. and S. E. Miller (2009), “Modern Uses of Electron Microscopy for Detection of Viruses”, *Clinical Microbiology Reviews*, 22 (4): 552–63.
Goldstein, J. and H. Yakowitz (1975), *Practical Scanning Electron Microscopy: Electron and Ion Microprobe Analysis*, New York: Plenum Press.
Goodman, P. S. and G. Pianigiani (2020), “Why Covid Caused Such Suffering in Italy’s Wealthiest Region”, *The New York Times*, November 19.
Goodsell, D. S. (2010), *The Machinery of Life*, 2nd ed., 2009 edition, New York: Copernicus.
Goodsell, D. S. (2012), “Illustrating the Machinery of Life: Viruses”, *Biochemistry and Molecular Biology Education*, 40 (5): 291–6.
Goodsell, D. S. (2016), “Quasisymmetry in Icosahedral Viruses”, *RCSB Protein Data Bank*.
Goodsell, D. S. (2020), “LASER Boston: ‘Shaping Biology & Behavior’”. Avaiable online at https://youtu.be/J1evuSAVRSs?si=GytlLnYisiiAvrkR.
Gorbalenya, A. E., S. C. Baker, R. S. Baric, R. J. de Groot, C. Drosten, A. A. Gulyaeva, B. L. Haagmans, C. Lauber, A. M. Leontovich, B. W. Neuman, D. Penzar, S. Perlman, L. L. M. Poon, D. V. Samborskiy, I. A. Sidorov, I. Sola, J. Ziebuhr, and Coronaviridae Study Group of the International Committee on Taxonomy of Viruses (2020), “The Species Severe Acute Respiratory Syndrome-Related Coronavirus: Classifying 2019-nCoV and Naming It SARS-CoV-2”, *Nature Microbiology*, 5 (4): 536–44.
Gordon, S. (1994), “The Generic Virus Writer”, *4th International Virus Bulletin Conference*.
Gordon, S. (2002), “What’s in a Name?” *SC magazine also published in Symantec White Pahes* (June).
Gordon, S. and R. Ford (2006), “On the Definition and Classification of Cybercrime”, *Journal of Computer virology*, 2: 13–20.
Goudsmit, J. (2004), *Viral Fitness: The Next SARS and West Nile in the Making*, New York: Oxford University Press.
Greensmith, J., A. Whitbrook and U. Aickelin (2010), “Artificial Immune Systems”, in M. Gendreau and J.-Y. Potvin (eds), *Handbook of Metaheuristics, International Series in Operations Research & Management Science*, 421–48, Boston, MA: Springer US.
Griffin, A. L. (2020), “Trustworthy Maps”, *Journal of Spatial Information Science*, 2020 (20): 5–19.
Grubaugh, N. D., J. T. Ladner, P. Lemey, O. G. Pybus, A. Rambaut, E. C. Holmes and K. G. Andersen (2019), “Tracking Virus Outbreaks in the Twenty-First Century”, *Nature Microbiology*, 4 (1): 10–19.
Guattari, F. (1989), “The Three Ecologies”, *New Formations*, (8): 131–47.
Guattari, F. (1995), *Chaosmosis: An Ethico-Aesthetic Paradigm*, Bloomington, IN: Indiana University Press.
Guattari, F. (1996), *Chaosophy-Soft Subversions*, New York: Semiotext(e).
Gupta, S. (2017), “The Big One Is Coming, and It’s Going to Be a Flu Pandemic”, *CNN*, Available online: http://www.cnn.com/2017/04/07/health/flu-pandemic-sanjay-gupta/index.html (accessed October 25, 2017).

Hall, S. (2018), "The West and the Rest: Discourse and Power", in D. Morley (ed), *Essential Essays, Volume 2*, 141–84, Durham: Duke University Press.

Halverson, C. (n.d.), "Biosociality: Where Diagnosis Intersects with Community ", Available online: http://hipporeads.com/biosociality-where-diagnosis-intersects-with-community/, (accessed August 9, 2017).

Haraway, D. (1988), "Situated Knowledges: The Science Question in Feminism and the Privilege of Partial Perspective", *Feminist Studies*, 14 (3): 575–99.

Haraway, D. J. (1992), "The Promises of Monsters: A Regenerative Politics for Inappropriate(d) Others", in L. Grossberg, C. Nelson and P. Treichler (eds), *Cultural Studies*, 295–337, New York London: Routledge.

Haraway, D. J. (1997), *Modest_Witness@Second _Millennium.FemaleMan© _Meets_OncoMouse™:Feminism and Technoscience*, New York: Routledge.

Herzberg, N. (2020), "Françoise Baylis: « La pandémie de Covid-19 nous offre un miroir grossissant de nos inégalités »", *Le Monde.fr*, June 2.

Hinterberger, A. and N. Porter (2015), "Genomic and Viral Sovereignty: Tethering the Materials of Global Biomedicine", *Public Culture*, 27 (2): 361–86.

Hoertel, N., M. Blachier, C. Blanco, M. Olfson, M. Massetti, M. S. Rico, F. Limosin and H. Leleu (2020), "A Stochastic Agent-Based Model of the SARS-CoV-2 Epidemic in France", *Nature Medicine*, 26 (9): 1417–21.

Holmdahl, I. and C. Buckee (2020), "Wrong but Useful—What Covid-19 Epidemiologic Models Can and Cannot Tell Us", *New England Journal of Medicine*, 383 (4): 303–5.

Hooke, R. (1780), *Microscopic Observations or, Dr. Hooke's Wonderful Discoveries by the Microscope, Illustrated by Thirty-three Copper-plates, Curiously Engraved: Whereby the Most Valuable Particulars in That Celebrated Author's Micrographia Are Brought Together in a Narrow Compass; and Intermixed, Occasionally, with Many Entertaining and Instructive Discoveries and Observations in Natural History*, printed for Robert Wilkinson, at No. 58, in Cornhill.

Hui, Y. (2015), "Towards a Relational Materialism A Reflection on Language, Relations and the Digital", *Digital Culture and Society*, 1 (1): 131–47.

Hurley, E. (2002), "The Virus Name Game", *Search Security*.

Hussein, H. (2020), "The Name Blame Game. A History of Inflammatory Illness Epithets", *Lapham's Quarterly*, 13 (3), Available online: https://www.laphamsquarterly.org/epidemic/maps/name-blame-game.

Iaconesi, S. (2013), "La Cura, an Open Source Cure for Cancer", *Big Data*, 1, Available online: http://online.liebertpub.com/doi/abs/10.1089/big.2013.0028.

ICTV (n.d.), *International Committee on the Taxonomy of Viruses—Introduction.*

ICTVdb (n.d.), *Virus Databases Online*. Available online at https://ictv.global/.

Jabr, F. (2020), "How Realistic Is Contagion? The Movie Doesn't Skimp on Science", *New Scientist*, April 6.

Jerram, L. (2017), "Glass Microbiology", *Issues in Science and Technology*, 33 (3), Available online: https://issues.org/?s=glass+microbiology.

Jerram, L. (n.d.), "Personal Website", Available online: www.lukejerram.com.

Johnston, S. F. (2018), "The Technological Fix as Social Cure-All: Origins and Implications", *IEEE Technology and Society Magazine*, 37 (1): 47–54.

Juliano, L. (2010), "Becoming Transreal: Micha Cardenas and Elle Mehrmand Mix First Life with Second Life", Center for the Study of Women, University of California Los Angeles, Available online: https://escholarship.org/uc/item/76b8b02k.

Kamel Boulos, M. N. and E. M. Geraghty (2020), "Geographical Tracking and Mapping of Coronavirus Disease COVID-19/Severe Acute Respiratory Syndrome Coronavirus 2 (SARS-CoV-2) Epidemic and Associated Events around the World: How 21st Century GIS Technologies Are Supporting the Global Fight against Outbreaks and Epidemics", *International Journal of Health Geographics*, 19 (1): 8.

Kamps, B. S. and G. Reyes-Terán (2006), "Influenza 2006", in B. S. Kamps and C. Hoffmann (eds), *Influenza Report 2006*. A medical text, 17–48, Flying Publisher.

Kaspersky Lab (n.d.), "MAP | Kaspersky Cyberthreat Real-Time Map", *MAP | Kaspersky Cyberthreat real-time map*, Available online: https://cybermap.kaspersky.com (accessed August 11, 2021).

Kay, L. E. (1995), "Who Wrote the Book of Life? Information and the Transformation of Molecular Biology, 1945–55", *Science in Context*, 8 (4): 609–34.

Kay, L. E. (1997), "Cybernetics, Information, Life: The Emergence of Scriptural Representations of Heredity", *Configurations*, 5 (1): 23–91.

Kay, L. E. (2000), *Who Wrote the Book of Life?: A History of the Genetic Code*, Stanford, CA: Stanford University Press.

Keeling, M. J. and K. T. D. Eames (2005), "Networks and Epidemic Models", *Journal of The Royal Society Interface*, 2 (4): 295–307.

Keller, E. F. (1995), *Refiguring Life*, New York: University of Columbia Press.

Keller, E. F. (2000), *The Century of the Gene*, Cambridge, MA: Harvard University Press.

Kelly, E. and S. J. Russell (2007), "History of Oncolytic Viruses: Genesis to Genetic Engineering", *Molecular Therapy*, 15 (4): 651–9.

Kephart, J. O., G. B. Sorkin and M. Swimmer (1997), "An Immune System for Cyberspace", *IEEE Computer Graphics and Applications*, 879–84.

Kephart, J. O., S. R. Chess and D. M. White (1993), "Computer and Epidemiology", *IEEE Spectrum*, 30 (5): 20–6.

Kermack, W. O., A. G. McKendrick and G. T. Walker (1927), "A Contribution to the Mathematical Theory of Epidemics", *Proceedings of the Royal Society of London. Series A, Containing Papers of a Mathematical and Physical Character*, 115 (772): 700–21.

Khazan, O. (2021), "Two Ways to Think About the New Mask Debate", *The Atlantic*, July 21.

Kirksey, E. (2020), *The Mutant Project: Inside the Global Race to Genetically Modify Humans*, New York: St. Martin's Press.

Koch, T. (2005), *Cartographies of Disease: Maps, Mapping, and Medicine*, Redlands, CA: ESRI Press.

Koch, T. (2011), *Disease Maps: Epidemics on the Ground*, Chicago; London: University of Chicago Press.

Krämer, K. (2017), "Cryo-EM: A Cold, Hard Look at Biology", *Chemistry World*, Available online: https://www.chemistryworld.com/feature/cryo-em-a-cold-hard-look-at-biology/3008131.article (accessed August 17, 2018).

Kroker, A. and M. Kroker (2006), "The New Biometric State", in *Born Again Ideology. Religion, Technology, Terrorism*, 67–82, Canada: CTheory Books.

Kuchment, A. (2011), *The Forgotten Cure: The Past and Future of Phage Therapy*, New York: Copernicus Books/Springer Science+Business Media.

Landecker, H. (2006), "Microcinematography and the History of Science and Film", *Isis*, 97 (1): 121–32.
Landecker, H. (2009), "Seeing Things: From Microcinematography to Live Cell Imaging", *Nature Methods*, 6 (10): 707–9.
Latour, B. (1983), "Give Me a Laboratory and I Will Raise the World", in M. Biagioli (ed), *The Science Studies Reader*, 258–75, New York: Routledge.
Latour, B. (1988), *Science in Action*, Cambridge, MA: Harvard University Press.
Latour, B. and S. Woolgar (1979), *Laboratory Life: The Social Construction of Scientific Facts*, Beverly Hills: Sage.
Lederberg, J. (2000), "Infectious History", *Science*, 287 (5464): 287–98.
Li, J. and P. Knickerbocker (2007), "Functional Similarities between Computer Worms and Biological Pathogens", *Computers & Security*, 26 (4): 338–47.
Li, J., S. Walker, J. Nie and X. Zhang (2019), "Experiments That Led to the First Gene-Edited Babies: The Ethical Failings and the Urgent Need for Better Governance", *Journal of Zhejiang University. Science. B*, 20 (1): 32–8.
Li, N., A. L. Molder and S. Yang (2022), "Visual Representations of SARS-CoV-2, Emotions, and Risk Perception of COVID-19", *Health Science Reports*, 5 (1): e496.
Li, Y. and H. L. Nicholson Jr. (2021), "When 'Model Minorities' Become 'Yellow Peril'—Othering and the Racialization of Asian Americans in the COVID-19 Pandemic", *Sociology Compass*, 15 (2): e12849.
Lin, H.-Y. (2003), *A Research of Computer Virus in the Visualization of 3D Computer Animation.*
Lin, P.-Y. (n.d.), "Pei-Ying Lin", Available online: http://peiyinglin.net (accessed February 21, 2021).
Liu, A. (2020), "'Chinese Virus,' World Market", *n+1*.
Longrigg, J. (1992), "Epidemics, Ideas and Classical Athenian Society", in T. Ranger and P. Slack (eds), *Epidemics and Ideas*, 21–44, Cambridge: University of Cambridge Press.
Lu, J. (2021), "Why Pandemics Give Birth to Hate: From Bubonic Plague to COVID-19", *NPR*, March 26.
Lucretius (2020), "The Nature of Plagues. A Roman Poet Revisits an Ancient Epidemic", *Lapham's Quarterly*.
Ludwig, M. (1995), *Computer Viruses, Artificial Life and Evolution*, Tucson, AZ: American Eagle publications.
Lukes, H. N. (2012), "Viral", *Women's Studies Quarterly*, 40 (1 & 2): 87–200.
Lynch, M. (1988), "The Externalized Retina: Selection and Mathematization in the Visual Documentation of Objects in the Life Sciences", *Human Studies*, 11 (2–3): 201–34.
Lynch, M. (2006), "The Production of Scientific Images: Vision and Re-Vision in the History, Philosophy, and Sociology of Science", in L. Pauwels (ed), *Visual Cultures of Science: Rethinking Representational Practices in Knowledge Building and Science Communication*, 26–40, Hanover, NH: Dartmouth College Press.
Lynteris, C. (2016a), "The Epidemiologist as Culture Hero: Visualizing Humanity in the Age of 'the Next Pandemic'", *Visual Anthropology*, 29 (1): 36–53.
Lynteris, C. (2016b), "The Prophetic Faculty of Epidemic Photography: Chinese Wet Markets and the Imagination of the Next Pandemic", *Visual Anthropology*, 29 (2): 118–32.

Lynteris, C. (2020), *Human Extinction and the Pandemic Imaginary*, Routledge studies in anthropology, Milton Park, Abingdon, Oxon: Routledge.
Macey, D. (2009), "Rethinking Biopolitics, Race and Power in the Wake of Foucault", *Theory, Culture & Society*, 26 (6): 186–205.
Mackenzie, A. (2014), "Multiplying Numbers Differently: An Epidemiology of Contagious Convolution", *Distinktion: Journal of Social Theory*, 15 (2): 189–207.
Mackenzie, L. S., R. Šebjanič, K. Żyniewicz, I. Burr Raty and D. Honorato (2021), "Staying in Touch: Case Study of Artistic Research during the COVID-19 Lock-Down", *Artnodes*.
Malik, D. J., I. J. Sokolov, G. K. Vinner, F. Mancuso, S. Cinquerrui, G. T. Vladisavljevic, M. R. J. Clokie, N. J. Garton, A. G. F. Stapley and A. Kirpichnikova (2017), "Formulation, Stabilisation and Encapsulation of Bacteriophage for Phage Therapy", *Advances in Colloid and Interface Science*, Recent Nanotechnology and Colloid Science Development for Biomedical Applications, 249: 100–33.
Manovich, L. (2001), *The Language of New Media*, Cambridge, MA: The MIT Press.
Manzoni, A. (1972), *The Betrothed*, The Penguin classics, London: Penguin Books.
Margulis, L. (1999), *Symbiotic Planet: A New Look at Evolution*, Revised ed., New York: Basic Books.
Margulis, L. and D. Sagan (2003), *Acquiring Genomes: A Theory of the Origin of Species*, Reprint edition, Princeton, NJ: Basic Books.
Martin, E. (1994), *Flexible Bodies: Tracking Immunity in American Culture—From the Days of Polio to the Age of Aids*, Boston: Beacon Press.
Martin, N. (2003), "Martin, Parasitic Media", *subsol*, Available online: http://subsol.c3.hu/subsol_2/contributors3/martintext.html (accessed February 13, 2024).
Marx, A. and F. Dessmann (2007), "The Wildlist is Dead, Long Live the Wildlist!", Virus Bulletin Conference, Vienna, Austria.
Massumi, B. (2002), *Parables for the Virtual: Movement, Affect, Sensation*, Durham, NC: Duke University Press.
Massumi, B. (2005), "Fear (The Spectrum Said)", *Positions*, 13 (1): 31.
Matzinger, P. (1994), "Tolerance, Danger, and the Extended Family", *Annual Review of Immunology*, 12 (1): 991–1045.
Matzinger, P. (2012), "The Evolution of the Danger Theory", *Expert review of clinical immunology*, 8 (4): 311–17.
McCormick, B. H. (1988), "Visualization in Scientific Computing", *ACM SIGBIO Newsletter*, 10 (1): 15.
McFall Ngai, A. (2017), "Noticing Microbial Worlds the Postmodern Synthesis in Biology", in A. L. Tsing, N. Bubandt, E. Gan and H. A. Swanson (eds), *Arts of Living on a Damaged Planet: Ghosts and Monsters of the Anthropocene*, 51–69, Minneapolis: University Of Minnesota Press.
McQullan, A. (2020), "Art, Science and a Pandemic: Laura Splan Returns for a Virtual Bioart Residency Focused on Sars-cov-2". Available online at https://sciencecenter.org/blog/art-science-and-a-pandemic-laura-splan-returns-for-a-virtual-bioart-residency-focused-on-sars-cov-2.
Milburn, C. (2002), "Nanotechnology in the Age of Posthuman Engineering: Science Fiction as Science", *Configurations*, 10 (2): 261–95.
Milliken, G. (2015), "Are Viruses Alive? New Evidence Says Yes Evolutionary History Suggests They Evolved from Ancient Cells", *Popular Science*, September.

Moelling, K. (2013), "What Contemporary Viruses Tell Us about Evolution: A Personal View", *Archives of Virology*, 158 (9): 1833–48.
Moelling, K. (2017), *Viruses: More Friends than Foes*, Singapore; Hackensack, NJ: World Scientific Publishing Co. Pte. Ltd.
Monmonier, M. (1996), *How to Lie with Maps*, Chicago: University of Chicago Press.
Monoyios, K. (2013), "You've Never Really Seen a Virus until You See This", *Scientific American Blog Network*.
Moran, M. H. (2017), "Missing Bodies and Secret Funerals: The Production of 'Safe and Dignified Burials' in the Liberian Ebola Crisis", *Anthropological Quarterly*, 90 (2): 399–421.
Morris, W. (2020), "For Me, Rewatching 'Contagion' Was Fun, Until It Wasn't", *The New York Times*, March 10.
Munster, A. (2006), *Materializing New Media: Embodiment in Information Aesthetics*, Dartmouth, NH: Dartmouth College Press.
Munster, A. (2013), *An Aesthesia of Networks: Conjunctive Experience in Art and Technology*, Cambridge, MA: The MIT Press.
Murdoch, T. B. and A. S. Detsky (2013), "The Inevitable Application of Big Data to Health Care", *JAMA*, 309 (13): 1351–52.
Murty, K. (2021), "Opinion: Mathematical Models Aren't Perfect, but They're a Key Tool in Fighting the Pandemic", *The Globe and Mail*, March 26.
Musu, C. (2020), "War Metaphors Used for COVID-19 Are Compelling but Also Dangerous", *The Conversation*.
Myers, N. (2015), *Rendering Life Molecular: Models, Modelers, and Excitable Matter*, Durham: Duke University Press.
Myers, N. (2014), "Rendering Machinic Life", in C. Coopmans, J. Vertesi, M. E. Lynch and S. Woolgar (eds), *Representation in Scientific Practice Revisited*, 153–76, Cambridge, MA: The MIT Press.
Nadwordny (2020), "Despite Mass Testing, University Of Illinois Sees Coronavirus Cases Rise", *NPR.org, Monday Report*, National Public Radio.
Nechvatal, J. (2002), "Voluptuous Viractualism Hermaphroditic Codes, Robotic Art and Immersive Excess", *CTheory*.
Nechvatal, J. (2011), *Immersion into Noise*, Ann Arbor: Open Humanities Press.
Nethercut, J. (2020), "Urbs/Orbis: Urban Cataclysm in Lucretius' De Rerum Natura", *Urbs/Orbis: Urban Cataclysm in Lucretius' De Rerum Natura*, 115–30, Leiden: De Gruyter.
Nguyen, N., O. Strnad, T. Klein, D. Luo, R. Alharbi, P. Wonka, M. Maritan, P. Mindek, L. Autin, D. S. Goodsell and I. Viola (2020), "Modeling in the Time of COVID-19: Statistical and Rule-Based Mesoscale Models", *Ieee Transactions on Visualization and Computer Graphics*, 27 (2): 722–32.
Norton Security (2020), "What Is a Honeypot? How It Can Lure Cyberattackers", Available online: https://us.norton.com/internetsecurity-iot-what-is-a-honeypot.html (accessed August 5, 2021).
O'Neil, C. (2017), *Weapons of Math Destruction: How Big Data Increases Inequality and Threatens Democracy*, First paperback edition, New York: Broadway Books.
O'Neil, C. (2020a), "10 Reasons to Doubt the Covid-19 Data", *Bloomberg.com*, April 13.
O'Neil, C. (2020b), "Meet the Covid Models That Are Running the World", *Bloomberg.com*, May 14.

Ornes, S. (2021), "Science and Culture: The Evolving Portrait of a Virus", *Proceedings of the National Academy of Sciences*, 118 (29): 1–4.
Otis, J. (2020), "History Need Not Repeat Itself When We Write the Journal of Our Plague Year | Jessica Otis", *The Guardian*, July 19.
Ou, C.-M. (2012), "Host-Based Intrusion Detection Systems Adapted from Agent-Based Artificial Immune Systems", *Neurocomputing*, Intelligent and Autonomous Systems, 88: 78–86.
Outbreak (1995), Action, Drama, Horror, [Film], Dir. Wolfgang Petersen, USA Warner Bros.
Pak, C. (2020), "Things and Trends: Images of COVID-19", *Medical Humanities*, Available online: https://blogs.bmj.com/medical-humanities/2020/04/22/things-and-trends-images-of-covid-19/ (accessed May 6, 2020).
Panese, F. (2006), "The Accursed Part of Scientific Iconography", in L. Pauwels (ed), *Visual Cultures of Science: Rethinking Representational Practices in Knowledge Building and Science Communication*, 63–89, Hanover, NH: Dartmouth College Press.
Panzeri, F., S. D. Paola and F. Domaneschi (2021), "Does the COVID-19 War Metaphor Influence Reasoning?", *PLOS ONE*, 16 (4): e0250651.
Parikka, J. (2005a), "Digital Monsters, Binary Aliens–Computer Viruses, Capitalism and the Flow of Information", *Fibreculture* (4).
Parikka, J. (2005b), "The Universal Viral Machine", *CTheory*.
Parikka, J. (2007), *Digital Contagions: A Media Archaeology of Computer Viruses*, New York: Peter Lang.
Pasveer, B. (2006), "Representing or Mediating: A History and Philosophy of X-Ray Images in Medicine", in L. Pauwels (ed), *Visual Cultures of Science: Rethinking Representational Practices in Knowledge Building and Science Communication*, 41–62, Hanover, NH: Dartmouth College Press.
Pauwels, L. (2006), "A Theoretical Framework for Assessing Visual Representational Practices in Knowledge Building and Science Communications", in L. Pauwels (ed), *Visual Cultures of Science: Rethinking Representational Practices in Knowledge Building and Science Communication*, 1–25, Hanover, NH: Dartmouth College Press.
Pearlman, A. (2017), "My Body, My Genes", *New Scientist*, 236 (3152): 22–3.
Phillips, L. (2014), "The Political Economy of Ebola", *Jacobin Magazine* 8, Available online: https://www.jacobinmag.com/2014/08/the-political-economy-of-ebola/.
Pizziconi, V., A. Garcia, B. Ramakrishna, W. Glaunsinger, A. Razdan, E. Ong and K. Hintze (1999), "Interactive Nano-Visualization for Science and Engineering Education", *Proceedings of the First Joint BMES/EMBS Conference. 1999 IEEE Engineering in Medicine and Biology 21st Annual Conference and the 1999 Annual Fall Meeting of the Biomedical Engineering Society*.
Poisot, T. (2020), "COVID-19 Models Demand an Abundance of Caution", *American Scientist*.
Prebus, A. F. (1998), "Events at the University of Alberta and the University of Toronto, Leading to the First North American Electron Microscope", *Micron*, 29 (4): 289–92.
Puig de la Bellacasa, M. (2017), *Matters of Care: Speculative Ethics in More than Human Worlds*, Posthumanities, Minneapolis: University of Minnesota Press.
Puigbò, P., Y. I. Wolf and E. V. Koonin (2013), "Seeing the Tree of Life behind the Phylogenetic Forest", *BMC Biology*, 11: 46.

Quammen, D. (2013), *Spillover: Animal Infections and the Next Human Pandemic*, Reprint edition, New York: WW Norton.
Rabinow, P. (1992), "Artificiality and Enlightment: From Sociobiology to Biosociality", in M. Biagioli (ed), *The Science Studies Reader*, 407–16, New York: Routledge.
Rabinow, P. (2008), "Artificiality and Enlightenment: From Sociobiology to Biosociality", in J. X. Inda (ed), *Anthropologies of Modernity*, 179–93, Blackwell Publishing Ltd.
Rabinow, P. and N. Rose (2006), "Biopower Today", *BioSocieties*, 1 (2): 195–217.
Racaniello, V. R. (2010), "Social Media and Microbiology Education", *PLOS Pathogens*, 6 (10): e1001095.
Racaniello, V. R. (2020), "Virology Lectures 2020 #1: What Is a Virus? MicrobeTV", Available online: https://www.youtube.com/watch?v=lj3NhPgOoX4.
Raiu, C. (2002), "A Virus by Any Other Name: Virus Naming Practices | *Symantec* Connect Community", *Symantec*, Available online: https://www.symantec.com/connect/articles/virus-any-other-name-virus-naming-practices (accessed October 10, 2019).
Raman, S. and R. Tutton (2010), "Life, Science, and Biopower", *Science, Technology & Human Values*, 35 (5): 711–34.
Rasmussen, N. (1996), "Making a Machine Instrumental: RCA and the Wartime Origins of Biological Electron Microscopy in America, 1940–1945", *Studies in History and Philosophy of Science Part A*, 27 (3): 311–49.
Rasmussen, N. (1999), *Picture Control: The Electron Microscope and the Transformation of Biology in America, 1940–1960*, Stanford, CA: Stanford University Press.
Rather, L. J. and J. B. Frerichs (1972), "On the Use of Military Metaphor in Western Medical Literature: The Bellum Contra Morbum of Thomas Campanell (1568–1639)", *Clio Medica*, 7 (3): 201–8.
Raymond, E. S. (1999), *The Cathedral and the Bazaar: Musings on Linux and Open Source by an Accidental Revolutionary*, 1st ed., Beijing: O'Reilly.
Raymond, J. R. (2020), "The Great Mask Debate: A Debate That Shouldn't Be a Debate at All", *WMJ: official publication of the State Medical Society of Wisconsin*, 119 (4): 229–39.
Reardon, S. (2014), "Phage Therapy Gets Revitalized", *Nature News*, 510 (7503): 15.
Regenmortel, M. H. V. van and B. W. J. Mahy (2004), "Emerging Issues in Virus Taxonomy", *Emerging Infectious Diseases*, 10 (1): 8–13.
Regenmortel, V. and C. M. Fauquet (2000), "Virus Taxonomy: Classification and Nomenclature of Viruses: Seventh Report of the International Committee on Taxonomy of Viruses", 1162, Academic Press.
Reilly, I. (2013), "From Critique to Mobilization: The Yes Men and the Utopian Politics of Satirical Fake News", *International journal of communication*, 7: 1243–64.
Reja, M. (2021), "Trump's 'Chinese Virus' Tweet Helped Lead to Rise in Racist Anti-Asian Twitter Content: Study", *ABC News*, Available online: https://abcnews.go.com/Health/trumps-chinese-virus-tweet-helped-lead-rise-racist/story?id=76530148 (accessed December 27, 2021).
Roach Pierson, R. (2007), "Elaine Whittaker: Review of Dreadful Visitations", *Mix*.
Roberts, P. (2004), "Virus Writers Wage Worm War. New Variants of Mydoom, Netsky, and Bagle Seen as Evidence of Escalating Feud", 3 March, Available online: http://www.pcworld.com/printable/article/id,115076/.

Roberts, S. (2020a), "Embracing the Uncertainties", *New York Times*.
Roberts, S. (2020b), "'The Pandemic Is a Prisoner's Dilemma Game'", *New York Times*.
Robins, K. (1996), *Into the Image: Culture and Politics in the Field of Vision*, London; New York: Routledge.
Robins, K. and F. Webster (1999), *Times of Technoculture: From Information Society to Virtual Life*, London; New York: Routledge.
Robbins, P. (2004), *Political Ecology: A Critical Introduction*, Malden, MA: Blackwell Pub.
Robinson, K. S. (2020), "The Coronavirus Is Rewriting Our Imaginations", *The New Yorker*, Available online: https://www.newyorker.com/culture/annals-of-inquiry/the-coronavirus-and-our-future (accessed May 4, 2020).
Roepstorff, K. (2017), *Influenza. Theatre of Glowing Darkness*, Venezia: Biennale di Venezia. 57. Esposizione Internazionale d'Arte.
Roff, R. J. (2008), "Preempting to Nothing: Neoliberalism and the Fight to de/Re-Regulate Agricultural Biotechnology", *Geoforum*, Rethinking Economy Agro-food activism in California and the politics of the possible Culture, nature and landscape in the Australian region, 39 (3): 1423–38.
Roof, J. (2007), *The Poetics of DNA*, Minneapolis: University Of Minnesota Press.
Roosth, S. (2013), "Biobricks and Crocheted Coral: Dispatches from the Life Sciences in the Age of Fabrication", *Science in Context*, 26 (1): 153–71.
Roosth, S. (2017), *Synthetic: How Life Got Made*, Chicago: The University of Chicago Press.
Rose, N. (2001), "The Politics of Life Itself", *Theory, Culture & Society*, 18 (6): 1–30.
Rosen, E. (2000), *The Anatomy of Buzz*, New York: Doubleday.
Ross, A. (1991), *Strange Weather. Culture, Science and Technology in the Age of Limits*, London; New York: Verso.
Rothman, K. J. (2002), *Epidemiology: An Introduction*, New York: Oxford University Press.
Rouse, J. (2004), "Barad's Feminist Naturalism", *Hypatia*, 19 (1): 142–61.
Roy, M., N. Moreau, C. Rousseau, A. Mercier, A. Wilson and L. Atlani-Duault (2020), "Ebola and Localized Blame on Social Media: Analysis of Twitter and Facebook Conversations during the 2014–2015 Ebola Epidemic", *Culture, Medicine, and Psychiatry*, 44 (1): 56–79.
Ruivenkamp, M. and A. Rip (2014), "Nanoimages as Hybrid Monsters", in J. Vertesi, M. E. Lynch, S. Woolgar and C. Coopmans (eds), *Representation in Scientific Practice Revisited*, 177–200, Cambridge, MA: The MIT Press.
Rushkoff, D. (1996), *Media Virus! Hidden Agendas in Popular Culture*, New York: Ballantine Books.
Ryan, F. (1997), *Virus X. Tracking the New Killer Plagues*, Boston; New York; Toronto: Little, Brown and co.
Sampson, T. (2004), "A Virus in Infospace: The Open Network and Its Enemies", *M/C media and Culture*, 7 (3), Available online: https://journal.media-culture.org.au/mcjournal/article/view/2368.
Sampson, T. (2005), "Dr. Aycock's Bad Idea. Is the Good Use of Computer Viruses Still a Good Idea?" *M/C media and Culture*, 8 (1), Available online: https://journal.media-culture.org.au/mcjournal/article/view/2314.
Sampson, T. D. (2012), *Virality: Contagion Theory in the Age of Networks*, Minneapolis: University Of Minnesota Press.

Sarkar, A. A. (2021), "New High-Resolution Imaging Technology Reveals COVID-19 Lung Pathology in Space and Time", *GEN—Genetic Engineering and Biotechnology News*.

Sattenspiel, L. and D. A. Herring (1998), "Structured Epidemic Models and the Spread of Influenza in the Central Canadian Subarctic", *Human Biology*, 70 (1): 91–115.

Schickore, J. (2009), "Test Objects for Microscopes" (accessed November 16, 2010).

Schneider, J. (2012), "Haraway's Viral Cyborg", *WSQ: Women's Studies Quarterly*, 40 (1): 294–300.

SciArt Initiative (2020), *LASER Boston: 'Shaping Biology & Behavior', Featured Talks by Amy Bucher, David Goodsell, Tobias Pforr, and Andreas Beerli*, LASER Boston.

Sepkowitz, K. (2009), "A Virus's Debut in a Doctor's Syringe", *New York Times*, D5.

Serres, M. (2007), *The Parasite*, Minneapolis: University of Minnesota Press.

Shah, S. (2017), *Pandemic: Tracking Contagions, from Cholera to Ebola and Beyond*, Reprint edition, New York: Picador.

Shao, C., G. L. Ciampaglia, O. Varol, A. Flammini and F. Menczer (2018), "The Spread of Fake News by Social Bots", *Nature Communications*, 9 (1): 4787.

Shao, C., G. L. Ciampaglia, O. Varol, K.-C. Yang, A. Flammini and F. Menczer (2018), "The Spread of Low-Credibility Content by Social Bots", *Nature Communications*, 9 (1): 4787.

Shieldings: Brighton Fringe Festival (2020), [documentary] Dir. Aristea Fotopoulou, Brighton Fringe Festival, video available at https://www.artdatahealth.org/shielding/.

Shapiro, P. (2020), "One Root Cause of Pandemics Few People Think About", *Scientific American Blog Network*, Available online: https://blogs.scientificamerican.com/observations/one-root-cause-of-pandemics-few-people-think-about/ (accessed May 8, 2022).

Shostak, S. (2010), "Marking Populations and Persons at Risk. Molecular Epidemiology and Environmental Health", in A. E. Clarke, L. Mamo, J. R. Fosket, J. R. Fishman and J. K. Shim (eds), *Biomedicalization: Technoscience, Health, and Illness in the U.S.*, 242–62, Durham: Duke University Press.

Siddell, S. (2018), "Why Virus Taxonomy Is Important", *Microbiology Today*, (Imaging).

Siggraph (1999), "History of Visualization", *Siggraph Education*, Available online: https://education.siggraph.org/static/HyperVis/visgoals/visgoal3.htm.

Sikora, S. (n.d.), "Balancing Art and Complexity: Joseph Nechvatal's Computer Virus Project", https://www.eyewithwings.net/nechvatal/Balancing/Balancing%20Art%20and%20Complex.htm.

Simmonds, P., M. J. Adams, M. Benkő, M. Breitbart, J. R. Brister, E. B. Carstens, A. J. Davison, E. Delwart, A. E. Gorbalenya, B. Harrach, R. Hull, A. M. Q. King, E. V. Koonin, M. Krupovic, J. H. Kuhn, E. J. Lefkowitz, M. L. Nibert, R. Orton, M. J. Roossinck, S. Sabanadzovic, M. B. Sullivan, C. A. Suttle, R. B. Tesh, R. A. van der Vlugt, A. Varsani and F. M. Zerbini (2017), "Consensus Statement: Virus Taxonomy in the Age of Metagenomics", *Nature Reviews Microbiology*, 15 (3): 161–8.

Singel, R. (2008), "Visualizing Viruses", *Wired*, May 12.

Singh, P. K. and A. Lakhotia (2002), "Analysis and Detection of Computer Viruses and Worms: An Annotated Bibliography", *ACM SIGPLAN Notices*, 37 (2): 2935.
Sivaramakrishnan, K. (2011), "The Return of Epidemics and the Politics of Global–Local Health", *American Journal of Public Health*, 101 (6): 1032–41.
Skormin, V. (2003), "Biological Approach to System Information Security (BASIS)", 72, Technical Report, Rome, New York: AIR FORCE RESEARCH LABORATORY INFORMATION DIRECTORATE, Available online: https://apps.dtic.mil/sti/tr/pdf/ADA420842.pdf.
Skormin, V., J. Moronski, D. L. McGee and D. H. Summerville (2003), "Biological Approach to System Information Security (BASIS): A Multi-Agent Approach to Information Security", *Multi-Agent Systems and Applications III, 3rd International Central and Eastern European Conference on Multi-Agent Systems, CEEMAS 2003*, 435–44.
Smelik, A. (2008), "Tunnel Vision: Inner, Outer and Virtual Space in Science Fiction Films and Medical Documentaries", in A. Smelik and N. Lykke (eds), *Bits of Life: Feminism at the Intersections of Media, Bioscience, and Technology*, 129–46, Seattle: University of Washington Press.
Smith, M. Roe (1994), "Technological Determinism in American Culture", in M. Roe Smith (ed), *Does Technology Drive History?: The Dilemma of Technological Determinism*, 1–36, Cambridge, MA: The MIT Press.
Spafford, E. H. (1994), "Computer Viruses as Artificial Life", *Artificial Life*, 1 (3): 249–65.
Splan, L. (2021), "Syndemic Sublime", *Visualizing the Virus*.
Stafford, B. M. (1993a), "Voyeur or Observer?: Enlightenment Thoughts on the Dilemmas of Display", *Configurations*, 1 (1): 95–128.
Stafford, B. M. (1993b), *Body Criticism: Imaging the Unseen in Enlightenment Art and Medicine*, Cambridge, MA: The MIT Press.
Stafford, B. M. (1996), *Good Looking: Essays on the Virtue of Images*, Cambridge, MA: The MIT Press.
Stengers, I. (2010), *Cosmopolitics I—University of Minnesota Press*, Minneapolis: University of Minnesota Press.
Stengers, I. (2011), *Cosmopolitics II—University of Minnesota Press*, Minneapolis: University of Minnesota Press.
Stewart, K. (2007), *Ordinary Affects*, Durham, NC: Duke University Press.
Stewart, K. (2010), "Worlding Refrains", in M. Gregg and G. J. Seigworth (eds), *The Affect Theory Reader*, 339–54, Durham: Duke University Press Books.
Subramani, M. R. and B. Rajagopalan (2003), "Knowledge Sharing and Influence in Online Networks via Viral Marketing", *Communications of the ACM*.
Svallingson, E. (2020), "To Visualise a Virus", *Karolinska Institutet Universitetsbiblioteket*.
Szor, P. (2005), *The Art of Computer Virus Research and Defense*, Upper Saddle River, NJ: Addison-Wesley.
Taub, A. (2020), "A New Covid-19 Crisis: Domestic Abuse Rises Worldwide", *The New York Times*, April 6.
Tavano, M. A. (2011), "Digital Brushstrokes: Diverse Techniques in Contemporary Digital Painting", The School of Arts and Sciences Rhode Island College.
Thacker, E. (2004), *Biomedia*, Minneapolis: University of Minnesota Press.
Thacker, E. (2005a), "Living Dead Networks", *Fibreculture* (4), Available online: https://four.fibreculturejournal.org/fcj-018-living-dead-networks/.

Thacker, E. (2005b), *The Global Genome: Biotechnology, Politics, and Culture*, 1st ed., Cambridge, MA: The MIT Press.
Thacker, E. (2009), "The Shadows of Atheology. Epidemics, Power and Life after Foucault", *Theory, Culture and Society*, 26 (6): 134–52.
Thatcher, J. (2014), "Big Data, Big Questions| Living on Fumes: Digital Footprints, Data Fumes, and the Limitations of Spatial Big Data", *International Journal of Communication*, 8: 19.
Thomas, A.-M. (2002), "It Came from Outer Space: The Virus, Cultural Anxiety, and Speculative Fiction", Doctoral Dissertation, Baton rouge: Louisiana State and Agricultural and Mechanical College.
Thomas, D. (2002), *Hacker Culture*, Minneapolis: University of Minnesota Press.
Thompson, D. (2017), "Mass Shootings in America Are Spreading Like a Disease", *The Atlantic*, November 6.
Thompson, D. (2020), "Hygiene Theater Is a Huge Waste of Time", *The Atlantic*, Available online: https://www.theatlantic.com/ideas/archive/2020/07/scourge-hygiene-theater/614599/ (accessed April 22, 2021).
Thucydides (1998), *The Peloponnesian War*, tran. S. Lattimore, Indianapolis: Hackett Publishing Company, Inc.
Tomes, N. (1999), *The Gospel of Germs. Men, Women and the Microbe in American Life*, Cambridge, MA: Harvard University Press.
TrendlabsResearch (2004), "The Sasser Event: History and Implications".
Trumbo, J. (1999), "Visual Literacy and Science Communication", *Science Communication*, 20 (4): 409–25.
Trumbo, J. (2000), "Essay: Seeing Science", *Science Communication*, 21 (4): 379–91.
Tufekci, Z. (2020), "Don't Believe the COVID-19 Models", *The Atlantic*, Available online: https://www.theatlantic.com/technology/archive/2020/04/coronavirus-models-arent-supposed-be-right/609271/ (accessed June 1, 2021).
Tufte, E. R. (1991), *Envisioning Information*, Cheshire, CT: Graphics Press.
Tufte, E. R. (2001), *The Visual Display of Quantitative Information*, Cheshire, CT: Graphics Press.
Tuhiwai Smith, P. Linda (2021), *Decolonizing Methodologies: Research and Indigenous Peoples*, London: Zed Books Ltd.
Turnbull, T. (2015), "Scientific Visualisation in Practice: Replicating Experiments at Scale", *Leonardo*, 48 (1): 72–3.
Turner, G. (1972), "Micrographia Historica: The Study of the History of the Microscope", *Proceedings of the Royai Microscopical Society* 7: 1220–49.
Twilley, N. (n.d.), "When a Virus Is the Cure", *The New Yorker*, Available online: https://www.newyorker.com/magazine/2020/12/21/when-a-virus-is-the-cure (accessed January 6, 2021).
University of Cambridge (2012), "DoITPoMS, Dissemination of IT for the Promotion of Materials Science", Online Instructional Manual, Available online: http://www.doitpoms.ac.uk/.
UPenn Arts & Science (2020). 60-Second Lectures in Quarantine: "Surviving Plagues Past and Present". Interview with David Barnes.
Van Den Eede, Y. (2011), "In Between Us: On the Transparency and Opacity of Technological Mediation", *Foundations of Science*, 16 (2–3): 139–59.
van der Tuin, I. and R. Dolphijn (2012), *New Materialism: Interviews & Cartographies*, Open University Press.

van Dijck, J. (2002), "Medical Documentary: Conjoined Twins as a Mediated Spectacle", *Media, Culture & Society*, 24 (4): 537–56.
van Dijck, J. (2005), *The Transparent Body: A Cultural Analysis of Medical Imaging*, Seattle: University of Washington Press.
van Dijck, J. (2006), "4 Picturizing Science. The Science Documentary as Multimedia Spectacle", in J. Willems and W. Göpfert (eds), *Science and the Power of TV*, 47–62, Amsterdam: VU University Press & Da Vinci Institute.
van Loon, J. (2002a), "A Contagious Living Fluid. Objectification and Assemblage in the History of Virology", *Theory, Culture and Society*, 19 (5/6): 107–24.
van Loon, J. (2002b), *Risk and Technological Culture: Towards a Sociology of Virulence*, London; New York: Routledge.
Villarreal, L. P. (2005), *Viruses and the Evolution of Life*, Washington, DC: ASM Press.
Villarreal, L. P. (2008), "Are Viruses Alive?", *Scientific American*, August 8. Available online at https://www.scientificamerican.com/article/are-viruses-alive-2004/.
Villarreal, L. P. (2016), "Persistent Virus and Addiction Modules: An Engine of Symbiosis", *Current Opinion in Microbiology*, Environmental microbiology * Special Section: Megaviromes, 31: 70–9.
Viral Narratives (2014), [Radio broadcast], WNYC On the Media, October 10.
Virilio, P. (2000), *The Information Bomb*, New York: Verso.
Viruses are Everywhere! (2011), [Radio broadcast] KERA RADIO, June 16.
Vonberg, J. (2017), "Scientists Win Nobel for Work to Visualize Biomolecules", *CNN*, Available online: https://www.cnn.com/2017/10/04/world/nobel-prize-chemistry-2017-cryo-electron-microsopy/index.html (accessed August 17, 2018).
Waal, A. de (2020), "New Pathogen, Old Politics", *Boston Review*, Text, Available online:http://bostonreview.net/science-nature/alex-de-waal-new-pathogen-old-politics (accessed July 17, 2020).
Wagner, E. K. and M. J. Hewlett (2004), *Basic Virology*, Malden, MA: Blackwell Science.
Wagner, M. (2017), "Defoe, Foucault, and the Politics of the Plague", *SEL Studies in English Literature 1500–1900*, 57 (3): 501–19.
Wald, P. (2008), *Contagious: Cultures, Carriers, and the Outbreak Narrative*, 1st ed., Durham: Duke University Press.
Wang, Y. (2020), "China Reports Second Death in Coronavirus Outbreak", *CTVNews*, Available online: https://www.ctvnews.ca/world/china-reports-second-death-in-coronavirus-outbreak-1.4771495 (accessed June 18, 2020).
Wasserman, H. (n.d.), "Cultural Factors Are behind Disinformation Pandemic: Why This Matters", *The Conversation*, Available online: http://theconversation.com/cultural-factors-are-behind-disinformation-pandemic-why-this-matters-141884 (accessed July 7, 2020).
Web Warriors (2009), [Film], Dir. Edward Peill, CBC Doc Zones.
Webb, P. (2005), *Essential Epidemiology: An Introduction for Students and Health Professionals*, New York: Cambridge University Press.
Webster, F., K. Rice and A. Sud (2020), "A Critical Content Analysis of Media Reporting on Opioids: The Social Construction of an Epidemic", *Social Science & Medicine*, 244: 112642.
Webster, M. and G. Malcolm (2008), "Classification of Computer Viruses Using a Theory of Affordances", *2nd International Workshop on the Theory of Computer Viruses (TCV 2007)*.

Weinraub, B. (1999), "'Blair Witch' Proclaimed First Internet Movie—Chicago Tribune", *Chicago Tribune*, August 17.
White, M. A. (2012), "Viral/Species/Crossing: Border Panics and Zoonotic Vulnerabilities", *Women's Studies Quarterly*, 40 (1 & 2): 117–37.
Whittaker, E. (2018), "Contained", *Elaine Whittaker*, Available online: https://www.elainewhittaker.ca/containedinstallation/ (accessed December 20, 2018).
Whittaker, E. (n.d.), "Elaine Whittaker's Webpage", Available online: http://www.etwhittaker.com/ (accessed October 8, 2012).
WHO (2008), "World Health Organization Outbreak Communication Planning Guide", Available online: https://www.afro.who.int/sites/default/files/2017-06/outbreak_com_plan_guide.pdf.
WHO (2021), "Ebola Virus Disease", Available online: https://www.who.int/news-room/fact-sheets/detail/ebola-virus-disease (accessed September 10, 2021).
WHO (2024), "Avian Influenza", Available online: https://www.who.int/westernpacific/wpro-emergencies/surveillance/avian-influenza.
WHO (2024), "Pandemic Influenza", Available online: https://www.who.int/teams/global-influenza-programme/public-health-preparedness.
WHO | Ebola Virus Disease (2023), *WHO*, Available online: http://www.who.int/mediacentre/factsheets/fs103/en/.
WHO- Health Topics (2020), "Infodemic", Available online: https://www.who.int/westernpacific/health-topics/infodemic (accessed September 29, 2021).
World Health Organization (WHO) (2024), Available online: https://www.who.int.
Wolfson, E. (2014), "Isolating Ebola-Affected Nations Could Worsen Outbreak, Experts Say", Available online: http://america.aljazeera.com/articles/2014/10/10/experts-isolatingebolaaffectednationscouldworsenoutbreak.html (accessed January 12, 2016).
Wong, A. (2015), "People with Leprosy Were Exiled There—Should It Be a Tourist Destination?" *The Atlantic*, Available online: https://www.theatlantic.com/health/archive/2015/05/when-the-last-patient-dies/394163/ (accessed August 17, 2021).
"*Worse than War": Health Workers on a Year of the Pandemic* (2021), [TV programme], AlJazeera, 10 March.
Yetiskin, E. (2014), "Paratactic Media and Social Networks: Emerging Forms of Resistance to Algorithmic Power in Artistic Practice", *Anglistica AION*, 18 (2): 107–25. ISSN: 2035-8504.
Yong, E. (2020a), "How the Pandemic Defeated America", *The Atlantic*.
Yong, E. (2020b), "Our Pandemic Summer", *The Atlantic*.
Yong, E. (2020c), "Why the Coronavirus Is So Confusing", *The Atlantic*.
Zhang, S. (2018), "A Biohacker Regrets Publicly Injecting Himself with CRISPR", *The Atlantic*, Available online: https://www.theatlantic.com/science/archive/2018/02/biohacking-stunts-crispr/553511/ (accessed May 13, 2022).
Zimmer, C. (2015), "Our Inner Viruses: Forty Million Years In the Making", *National Geographic Magazine*.
Zimmer, C. (2016), "Scientists Unveil New 'Tree of Life'", *The New York Times*, April 11.
Zimmer, C. (2020), "The Coronavirus Unveiled", *The New York Times*, October 9.
Zimmer, C. (2021), *A Planet of Viruses: Third Edition*, Chicago; London: University of Chicago Press.

Index